Praise for *We'll Fight It Out Here*

T0247742

"This inspiring, engaging, and informativ
systemic barriers African Americans faced but also the extraordinary
agency Black leaders demonstrated in overcoming some of these obstacles. At a time when health disparities have gained national attention, this is a story of solutions and hope, beautifully told."
—Kenneth M. Ludmerer, MD, Washington University
    in St. Louis, author of *Let Me Heal: The Opportunity*
    to Preserve Excellence in American Medicine

"*We'll Fight It Out Here* is a David and Goliath legislative story of how a
small and dedicated group of health professionals battled to eliminate
health disparities and push through Congress legislation that opened
up first-rate medical care to African Americans. It is a historical gem of
how participants in the legislative process in Washington can be persuaded to do the right thing for those in greatest need."
—Joseph A. Califano Jr., former US Secretary of
    Health Education and Welfare

"This is an essential work on American medical history and its place in
the fight for racial justice. The story is dramatic and lucid. The book
should be mandatory reading for college courses and for anyone interested in America's ongoing search for racial equality. It represents a
milestone in writing on medical history and should be part of the core
knowledge of all those who care about equitable and human health care."
—Augustus A. White III, MD, PhD, Harvard Medical School,
    author of *Seeing Patients: A Surgeon's Story of Race and*
    Medical Bias

"An amazing story of grit, determination, and perseverance to advance
Black and minority-serving health institutions. To have a more just and
equitable nation, more attention and support must be given to the cher-
ished institutions that compose the Association of Minority Health Professions Schools."
—Wayne J. Riley, MD, MPD, President, SUNY Downstate
    Health Sciences University

WE'LL FIGHT IT OUT HERE

We'll Fight It Out Here

A History
of the Ongoing Struggle
for Health Equity

DAVID CHANOFF

AND LOUIS W. SULLIVAN

With a New Foreword
from Daniel E. Dawes

JOHNS HOPKINS UNIVERSITY PRESS | BALTIMORE

Johns Hopkins Paperback edition, 2024
2 4 6 8 9 7 5 3 1

Johns Hopkins University Press
2715 North Charles Street
Baltimore, Maryland 21218
www.press.jhu.edu

Library of Congress Cataloging-in-Publication Data

Names: Chanoff, David, author. | Sullivan, Louis Wade, 1933– author.
Title: We'll fight it out here : a history of the ongoing struggle
for health equity / David Chanoff and Louis W. Sullivan.
Description: Baltimore: Johns Hopkins University Press, 2022. |
Includes bibliographical references and index.
Identifiers: LCCN 2021063003 | ISBN 9781421444642 (hardcover) |
ISBN 9781421444659 (ebook)
Subjects: LCSH: Association of Minority Health Professions Schools
(U.S.)—History. | African Americans in medicine. | Racism in
medicine—United States. | Discrimination in medical
education—United States. | African Americans—Medical care—
Social aspects—United States. | Discrimination in medical care—
United States. | Health and race—United States. | Health services
accessibility—United States.
Classification: LCC R695 .C43 2022
LC record available at https://lccn.loc.gov/2021063003

A catalog record for this book is available from the British Library.

ISBN 978-1-4214-5044-5 (paperback)

Special discounts are available for bulk purchases of this book. For more information,
please contact Special Sales at specialsales@jh.edu.

To the Memory of Louis Stokes
Health Care Champion for the Poor and Underserved

CONTENTS

Foreword to the Paperback Edition ix
Preface xv
Timeline xxiii

1 The Nadir 1

2 The Response 18

3 Abraham Flexner and the
Black Medical Schools 36

4 AMHPS: The Founding 48

5 The Heckler Report 72

6 Landmark Legislation 84

7 AMHPS and the Secretary 103

8 The Office of Minority Health 120

9 The Center for Minority Health
and Health Disparities 142

10 A National Institute 165

11 A Common Mission 190

Afterword 212

Acknowledgments 219
Notes 223
Index 231
Photographs follow page 138

We'll Fight It Out Here tells the extraordinary story of a little-known group of minority health professions schools that almost single-handedly brought disparities and inequitable care to the public's attention and spearheaded legislation benefiting underserved populations, white and Brown as well as Black. When the Association of Minority Health Professions Schools (AMHPS) was founded in 1976, health care inequities were not part of mainstream public health thinking. Many, even among practitioners and clinical scientists, regarded the idea as little more than imaginative fiction. But the heads of the four Black health schools (Morehouse School of Medicine, Meharry Medical College, Xavier University College of Pharmacy, and Tuskegee University College of Veterinary Medicine) who had initially constituted the new association knew differently. America's Black population was suffering levels of morbidity and mortality that far surpassed disease and death rates among white Americans. Black people lived shorter lives than white people. Black maternal and infant death rates were especially alarming. Cancer, vascular and heart disease, diabetes, and other severe illnesses were less treated and more lethal among Blacks than whites. The number of African American doctors and other health practitioners was woefully inadequate. Stark inequities prevailed in almost every field of medicine.

In 1983 the AMHPS presented a report on Black health to President Ronald Reagan's secretary of health and human services,

Margaret Heckler. It was the first time that comprehensive figures on health disparities had been compiled and documented. Secretary Heckler appointed a committee to investigate, and two years later she issued the *Report of the Secretary's Task Force on Black and Minority Health*. "To bring the health of minorities to the level of all Americans," the report declared, "efforts of monumental proportions were needed." The Heckler Report (as it came to be known) declared that America's government had an obligation to address the health care needs of the country's minorities—"which it had not done," authors Chanoff and Sullivan write, "since Reconstruction, more than a hundred years earlier, and little enough then."

The Heckler Report laid the groundwork for a series of landmark health bills that drew bipartisan support, enhancing the minority schools' research and clinical programs, assuring an increasing flow of minority physicians and medical scientists, and confronting the inequities that were then and still are plaguing American health care. Almost all the health bills that became law prior to Obamacare were initiated and shepherded through the legislative process by the AMHPS and its advocacy arm.

Perhaps the most significant achievement of the AMHPS was the establishment of the Office for Minority Health of the National Institutes of Health, today the Institute for Minority Health and Health Disparities. The Institute and its predecessors, the Office, then the Center for Minority Health, have played a lead role in spotlighting minority health issues and health inequities that are now so prominent in the national conversation. In essence, the AMHPS established a new framework for thinking about health care and its social, political, and economic consequences, bringing these subjects out of the shadows and onto the national stage. Disparate care, we know now, is ingrained in our health system, knowledge that has allowed us to take ameliora-tive measures and confront the challenges still ahead.

We'll Fight It Out Here paints a vivid picture of this legislative history and the until now obscure association of minority schools that drove it. Legislative chronicles can be powerful soporifics, but this history has drama, tension, and heroes and villains. The AMHPS threaded its way through the Reagan years of slashed budgets, Newt Gingrich's scorched-earth assault on everything deemed welfare, and the fierce partisan warfare that upended so much of American political life for so many years now. It's a his-tory full of surprises: rock-ribbed Republicans like Georgia's Charlie Norwood, who sponsored groundbreaking health legis-lation; long-term Congressman Jimmy Quillen from Tennessee, who knocked down opposition from archconservatives in his own party; hard-right Republicans Mack Mattingly and Thad Cochran, who filibustered to preserve minority health school fund-ing that would have died in Democratic attacks on appropriations. The way Democrat and Republican coalitions came together to further minority health issues provides some encouragement to hopes that even in periods of heightened antagonism, certain issues can generate accord—a needed and welcome reminder in dark political times.

The history that *We'll Fight It Out Here* recounts includes a discussion of how AMHPS-driven legislation, designed to help Black institutions and Black health care consumers, has spread its wings over institutions that serve equally disadvantaged pop-ulations, including white, Hispanic, Native American, and other populations. "The mostly unseen workings of the democratic ethos," as the authors describe it, are "almost inevitably spread-ing its penumbra over different groups of the society's marginal-ized and disregarded." It was at the insistence of Senator Robert

Byrd of West Virginia that the Office for Minority Health became the Center (now the Institute) for Minority Health *and Health Disparities*. The act establishing the Institute described "other populations with health disparities," which initially referred only to the sociologically disadvantaged and underserved rural populations of West Virginia and other Appalachian states but has since spread its "penumbra" farther.

We'll Fight It Out Here presents a wealth of little-known but important historical information and insight essential to understanding the ongoing problem of health inequities. The first three chapters in particular should be required reading for everyone interested in the evolution of Black medicine and medical institutions. These chapters treat the slow and painful struggle of Black physicians entering the world of mainstream American medicine, from Revolutionary times to the early twentieth century, when the Carnegie Foundation's Flexner Report led to the demise of over half of all American and Canadian medical schools, including five of the seven Black institutions that existed then, which left Howard and Meharry as the only minority survivors of Flexner's brutally straightforward evaluations.

These chapters tell the story of the nadir of Black health following the Civil War's emancipation of more than four million enslaved persons, creating massive refugee crises not only in health but also in other necessities of life, such as food, clothing, shelter, and education—a massive uprooting of people, as one government health official put it, into "extreme destitution and suffering." *We'll Fight It Out Here* describes the struggle of the Black community (along with white allies) to respond to the postwar chaos by building its own health infrastructure out of scant resources in the face of entrenched racial antipathy. Howard University College of Medicine and Meharry Medical College had their origins in Freedmen's Bureau funding, though the character, student bodies, and impact of the two schools differed markedly. Meharry's founding story is especially interesting and little known outside Meharry circles. Excluded from membership in local and regional medical societies (essential for hospital affiliation and advanced training), Black physicians created their own societies. Black physicians likewise founded hospitals and nursing schools to serve the African American population and provide training and practice facilities for Black doctors and nurses when mainstream institutions' doors were closed to them. In 1895 twelve leading Black physicians banded together to found the National Medical Association as a counterpart to the whites-only American Medical Association, which only changed its bylaws to prohibit racial discrimination in 1968 and did not apologize for its history of prejudice until 2008.

A striking aspect of the AMHPS's efforts is the continuity from early Black doctors to modern-era physicians such as Louis Sullivan, David Satcher, Donna Christensen, Regina Benjamin, and others. Leading figures from among the earliest cohort of African American physicians often carried on their medical practices simultaneously with political activity. James McCune Smith, Martin Robison Delany, and John Swett Rock were fierce abolitionists, outraged by slavery and the rigid constrictions imposed on free Blacks as well. Smith and Delany were close colleagues of Frederick Douglass and Swett Rock, a physician who later became a lawyer and was the first African American admitted to practice before the Supreme Court. A direct line connects their fight for equal rights with Sullivan, Satcher, Christensen, Benjamin, and the other AMHPS leaders who created and worked political levers to counteract the prejudice and relegation that stand behind so many of the devastating health disparities that still beset America's Black community. *We'll Fight It Out Here* allows us to see a pivotal piece of America's racial history as it has rarely been depicted.

Daniel E. Dawes, JD, author of *The Political Determinants of Health*; founding dean of the School of Global Health at Meharry Medical College

A hundred and thirty years before the COVID-19 pandemic cast its harsh light on the deadly reality of racialized health disparities, the leading statistician of the Progressive Era set himself the task of determining why it was that African Americans were more prone to serious disease than white Americans. Why were African Americans sicker than whites, Frederick Hoffman asked. Why did they die at faster rates and live shorter lives?

Since childhood Hoffman had been obsessed by numbers, and since his emigration from Germany to the United States at age nineteen he had been equally obsessed by the differences between white and Black Americans. In 1896, working as a statistician for the Prudential Insurance Company, he released a book-length study, *Race Traits and Tendencies of the American Negro*, a compendium of data and analysis detailing the reasons for the difference between the health of Blacks and whites. The study was published by the American Economic Association in two successive issues of its official journal, which attested to the work's credibility and helped make *Race Traits* the most influential social science document of its time. In mathematically precise terms Hoffman conveyed a devastating picture of Black health in America. The data, he said, pointed to only one conclusion: the Black race was on a one-way path to extinction.

His conclusion, Hoffman declared, was based wholly on incontrovertible facts and numbers. Prejudice had no part in it. Having come to America as an immigrant, he had never been exposed to or influenced by the racist assumptions so prevalent in his adopted country. "Being of foreign birth, a German," he wrote, "I was fortunately free from a personal bias."[1]

Hoffman's study was widely considered a triumph of objective statistical analysis. But there were detractors as well. Some of his opponents, including the famed Black sociologist and historian W. E. B. Du Bois, pointed out that his analysis was defective on various counts and, despite Hoffman's claims, unscientific. Hoffman had not compared Black mortality rates with those of similarly impoverished white groups. He had neglected to consider the weight of social determinants in the mortality numbers—poor nutrition, housing, and clothing; subpar education; and job discrimination. The high Negro death rate, Du Bois explained, was attributable to the differences between Black and white conditions of life. And even given those circumstances, the high death rate didn't threaten the extinction of the race.

Hoffman answered that "it is not in the conditions of life, but in the race traits and tendencies that we find the cause of excessive mortality." Black people, he said, "had a race proclivity to disease and death." They were, simply put, biologically inferior to whites, and that inferiority was leading them inevitably down the road to racial collapse.[2] "The Indian," Hoffman wrote, "is on the verge of extinction . . . the African will surely follow him."[3]

Time proved Hoffman's extinction thesis a myth. African Americans did not die out. On the contrary, their numbers grew. The 1910 census found that the 8.8 million African Americans counted in 1900 had, in ten years, grown to 9.8 million, an increase of 11 percent. Du Bois was right, Hoffman wrong.

But although African Americans were not doomed to extinction, the numbers Hoffman had based his calculations on were not by themselves misleading. It wasn't the numbers that were wrong; it was the racist framework that dictated his flawed methodology. In

1900 the Black mortality rate was 70 percent higher than the white. White men and women could expect to live many years longer than their Black counterparts. Black infant mortality rates were especially alarming: 371 Black babies died out of every thousand live births, compared with 158 white babies. Savannah, Georgia, had the highest rate, an astonishing 409 Black infant deaths per thousand live births. Du Bois called it "the slaughter of the innocents."[4]

Among the social and environmental reasons that Du Bois and others noted for these disparities, one of the most glaring was the lack of medical care available for African Americans, most especially in the rural South, home to almost 90 percent of the Black population. In 1895, the year before Hoffman's *Race Traits* was published, there were approximately nine hundred Black doctors in the country,[5] many practicing in isolated rural areas with little or no access to contemporary developments in medical science and no hospitals to which they could admit patients. No Southern medical school accepted Black students; of the few schools in the North that would even consider applications from African Americans, it was rare for a Black student to gain admission. A small flow of doctors emerged from the seven Black medical schools that existed at the turn of the century, most of which were threadbare institutions perched perilously on the verge of collapse. Only two of the seven, Howard Medical School in Washington, DC, and Meharry Medical College in Nashville, Tennessee, survived the stringent evaluations of the Carnegie Foundation's 1910 Flexner Report, a review of all medical schools in the country by Abraham Flexner, an educator and reformer.

As the twentieth century unfolded, the number of Black health practitioners increased but not in sufficient numbers, particularly in the South, and not nearly enough to begin decreasing the stark differences between the health of white and Black Americans. By the end of the 1970s the percentage of African Americans among the nation's health professionals had not increased over what it had been in 1910. The continuing, extreme shortage of Black physicians and other health practitioners meant that three-quarters of a century after Hoffman published his report, the African American death rate, infant mortality rate, and life span were still shockingly discordant with national norms.

In 1975 Meharry and Howard, the two Black medical schools that survived the Flexner Report, were joined by a third, the newly established Morehouse School of Medicine. In financial terms, Howard, which enjoyed an annual federal subsidy legislated in 1879, was relatively stable; but Meharry was in dire straits, and Morehouse, launched on a shoestring, desperately needed funding to ensure its survival and build its start-up programs. In the late 1970s Morehouse and Meharry, together with Xavier University College of Pharmacy in New Orleans and Tuskegee College of Veterinary Medicine in Alabama, formed a coalition to give their institutions a combined voice in advocating for federal funding. Each of them was motivated by need (Howard, buoyed by its federal subsidy, did not join). Together, they knew that the failure or deterioration of their institutions would have severe consequences for an African American community already suffering illness and death at barely tolerable levels.

In 1983 the original group of Black health professions schools, along with the colleges of pharmacy of Florida A&M University and Texas Southern University, and the new Charles R. Drew University of Medicine and Science incorporated their coalition as the Association of Minority Health Professions Schools (AMHPS). In their approach to the Reagan administration, they underscored the critical role their institutions played in training the African American doctors, dentists, and pharmacists so essential to the health of the minority community. They spelled out the fragile state of their institutional resources and the country's history of ignoring and dismissing minority health issues. They identified specific areas of great concern—cancer, cardiac health, and maternal health and obstetrics—emphasizing the lack of access to health care of any kind, a situation prevalent in both rural and urban Black communities. They argued that America's government had an obligation to address the health needs of the country's minorities—which it had not done since Reconstruction, more than a hundred years earlier, and little enough then.

In 1983 four AMHPS leaders presented their case to President Ronald Reagan's secretary of health and human services, Margaret Heckler. Heckler was a moderate Republican from Massachusetts, but the four leaders—Louis W. Sullivan, founding dean of Morehouse; David Satcher, president of Meharry; Walter Bowie, dean at Tuskegee; and Alfred Haynes, president of Drew—weren't optimistic that their presentation would come to anything. The Reagan budgets had been slashed in virtually every area except defense. Programs supporting Black and other needy medical students had been crippled, as had other social programs important to the Black community. Heckler could be a possible conduit to funding legislation for the Black schools, if she could be won over. But given the political climate, they weren't sure that would happen. The chances were good that the secretary would give them a polite hearing, then disregard their appeal.

The meeting with Heckler was friendly but inconclusive. Heckler promised to read the 120-page AMHPS white paper and get back to them, but that sounded as if it might be the polite brushoff they half expected. When months passed with no response, it seemed clear their argument had fallen on stony ground. Then, a year after their meeting, they did hear back. Heckler had appointed a committee to examine their concerns.

Another year passed before the committee report was ready. Heckler published it in 1985 as the *Report of the Secretary's Task*

Force on Black and Minority Health. "There was," she said in her foreword, "a continuing disparity in the burden of death and illness experienced by Blacks and other minority Americans." The report, she hoped, would "mark the beginning of the end of the health disparity that has, for so long, cast a shadow on . . . the American track record of ever improving health." It was the first explicit federal government acknowledgment that disparities in health existed and that they constituted a national problem.

Circulated through Congress, the Heckler Report (as it became known) served as the driving force behind a string of extraordinary legislative successes that strengthened the finances of minority schools and bolstered their clinical, research, and student recruitment efforts. The hearings on these minority health bills had an additional effect: they engendered an awareness of the severity of minority health problems in Congress, where before a kind of willful ignorance had prevailed. However, although the congressional health and appropriations committees engaged with these issues, there was still little public understanding of the severity of minority health deficits or their impact on the nation's health generally.

The AMHPS white paper had precipitated the Heckler Report and had served as a guide for Secretary Heckler's task force. The lobbying efforts of the AMHPS leadership had figured prominently in introducing the minority health bills and achieving their success. As the Reagan administration gave way to the Bush administration and then succeeding administrations, AMHPS was primarily responsible for the establishment in 2000 of a National Institutes of Health Center (elevated to an NIH Institute in 2010) of Minority Health and Health Disparities. A small organization with a modest budget, AMHPS operated outside the range of public visibility, yet it brought about major changes in the way the country's medical establishment viewed Black and other minority health problems.

~

Even with the congressional successes, it took years to reshape the perspectives of doctors and medical scientists to understand the magnitude and pervasiveness of health disparities, and only slowly did this understanding seep into the public conversation about bias in the nation's health system. But suddenly, in the winter and spring of 2020, the COVID-19 pandemic brought the disparities between the health of minority groups and white Americans into the bright light of day.

Through the pandemic's first year, the African American death rate was 270 percent above the white rate, and hospitalizations among African Americans were 370 percent higher. These are numbers that recall the morbidity and mortality statistics first gathered by Frederick Hoffman at the end of the nineteenth century. Hoffman's accounting back then was done with racist intent. His objective was to prove for the benefit of the Prudential Insurance Company, his employer, that African Americans presented higher risks than whites, which justified both raising premiums and even excluding them from buying insurance. There was no sense then that the pronounced health deficits of the Black population should occasion any kind of ameliorative steps.

But times change. Since 1985 with the AMHPS-inspired Heckler Report, a significant amount of legislation has passed, addressing one dimension or another of the problem. NIH has recognized the severity of minority health issues by establishing an institute dedicated to improving them. Congressional champions have emerged to lead the legislative battles: Louis Stokes, Warren Magnuson, Ted Kennedy, Bill Frist, John Porter, Tom Harkin, and Arlen Specter in the past, and in today's Congress, Cory Booker, Tim

Scott, and others. At the same time, AMHPS played a key role in highlighting the ability of African American medical leaders to precipitate and channel a new course of events in the development of American health care. In this sense the coalition of Black health professions schools paralleled the Black political coalition that came together in 1971 as the Congressional Black Caucus, which worked in tandem with AMHPS on much of its legislative agenda. The two coalitions marked the new exercise of Black empowerment that was taking place in different sectors of American life in the wake of the civil rights laws.

～

We'll Fight It Out Here takes a close look at the work of the Association of Minority Health Professions Schools as a leader in congressional battles to address the racial inequities that help relegate American health care to the lowest rung among the world's developed nations.

The congressional battleground is replete with drama and confrontation, alliances and showdowns. It has its own towering figures, both heroes and villains. It is on the congressional stage that we can most vividly see the march toward the national ideal of equality and the counterthrust of tenacious racism. It is on this stage too that the stark revelations of the COVID-19 pandemic about inequities in health care will play out, either to further the inertia that afflicts our attempts to remedy these disparities or to trigger new, meaningful initiatives toward closing the nation's long-standing racial health divide.

TIMELINE

1977—AMHPS founded

1978 (passed)/1981 (funded)—Title III, Section 326, Strengthening Historically Black Graduate Institutions
Extended government support for undergraduate Historically Black Colleges and Universities to include graduate institutions, first for medical school programs and later for graduate programs in a variety of disciplines.

1983—AMHPS White Paper, *Blacks and the Health Professions in the '80s: A National Crisis and a Time for Action*

1985—Heckler Report, *Report of the Secretary's Task Force on Black and Minority Health*

1985—HHS Secretary Margaret Heckler initiates the process to establish the Office of Minority Health under a deputy assistant secretary (the office is created the following year)

1986—Research Centers in Minority Institutions (RCMI) program passed as part of appropriations bill for HHS
Funding for research infrastructure at traditionally Black institutions.

1987—Title VII, Excellence in Minority Health Education and Care Act
Makes grants available to minority institutions that have provided leadership in producing practitioners for

underserved populations. Initially intended for predominantly Black institutions, the scope expanded to include
Hispanic-serving and Native American–serving schools.

1988—**NIH grant for establishing biomedical symposia on
health care careers for minority high school and college
students**
Grants were made through 1997.

1989—**President George H. W. Bush appoints Louis W. Sullivan
as HHS secretary**

1990—**HHS Secretary Sullivan establishes the NIH Office of
Minority Programs**
This becomes the National Center on Minority Health and
Health Disparities in 2000.

1990—**Title I, Disadvantaged Minority Health Improvement Act**
Funding for minority schools to offer scholarships to needy
students.

1993—**NIH Revitalization Act**
Mandated equity regarding the enrollment of women and
minorities in clinical research trials.

2000—**The Minority Health and Health Disparities Research
and Education Act**
Established the NIH National Center on Minority Health
and Health Disparities, raising the Office of Minority
Programs to a Center, with its own budget and grantmaking authority.

2010—**Elevation of the Center on Minority Health and Health
Disparities to an NIH Institute through an amendment to
the Affordable Care Act**

WE'LL FIGHT IT OUT HERE

CHAPTER 1

The Nadir

Primus Manumit's slave name is not recorded. His original African name is not known. Manumit lived in Windsor, Connecticut, in the latter part of the eighteenth century, an enslaved man owned by Dr. Alexander Wolcott. He assisted the doctor in his medical practice for many years before being freed, taking an appropriate new name, and establishing himself as a physician in his own right, with what we are told was a "considerable practice."[1] The substantial two-story house where he lived and saw patients is still standing. As far as we know, Manumit was the first African American accepted by white society as a physician.

Manumit practiced during the Revolutionary War. Another, better-known Black physician of that period was James Derham (or Durham). Enslaved upon birth in Philadelphia in 1762, Derham was owned by and assisted a series of physicians; the last one, Dr. Robert Dow of New Orleans, gave him his freedom and helped him set up an independent practice. Benjamin Rush, the eminent Philadelphia doctor, abolitionist, and signer of the Declaration of Independence, wrote about Derham, "I have conversed with him upon most of the acute and epidemic diseases . . . and was pleased to find him perfectly acquainted with the modern simple mode of practice in those diseases. I expected to have suggested some new medicines to him, but he suggested many more to me."[2]

Manumit and Derham were the first of the Black physicians who began to penetrate the world of American medicine toward the turn of the eighteenth and nineteenth centuries. Among those who followed closely after them were Martin Robison Delany and James McCune Smith. Delany was apprentice-trained in Pittsburgh under the supervision of several prominent white doctors. He later spent a semester at Harvard Medical School, before being forced to withdraw, along with two Black classmates, after a protest by a group of white students who complained that the presence of Black students was "highly detrimental to the interests and welfare of the institution."[3] Delany and his two colleagues were joined in their forced exodus from Harvard by Harriet Kezia Hunt, the first woman to gain admittance. "Racism and patriarchy," as one commentator put it, "went hand in hand."

Smith, like Delany, had been turned down by several American medical schools, but abolitionist friends provided the financial support for him to attend Glasgow University, whose medical school was one of Europe's most prominent. Smith earned his bachelor's, master's, and medical degrees there, graduating near the top of his medical school class, and then completing an internship in Paris.

Delany and Smith would have been exceptional in any period. Both were uncommonly intelligent, erudite, articulate—doctors but also courageous public figures. Both were determined, outspoken abolitionists and natural allies. And yet they found themselves on different sides of *the* essential question facing free Black Americans prior to the Civil War.

That question was emigration. For free Blacks in the prewar period, emigration decidedly did not mean the Liberian colonization scheme, despised by many as a ploy to remove African Americans from their homes for the benefit of whites who refused to accept them as fellow citizens. "We live here—have lived here—have a right to live here, and mean to live here," Frederick Douglass wrote in *The North Star*, his first newspaper.[4] Liberian colonization was a plan designed by whites and controlled by whites, for the benefit of whites. Emigration, on the contrary, was a Black response to the intolerable conditions of even free Black life in America, a proposal that American Blacks should found their own country in some foreign place, preferably Africa, the hereditary homeland, or instead another receptive region such as South America.

The "Back to Africa" idea had been in circulation since the late eighteenth century and began to grow into a movement in the first half of the nineteenth. A number of Northern Black leaders advocated the return, especially after the fugitive slave law passed in 1850, which provoked outrage and defiance among Northern Blacks as well as among white abolitionists. By 1852 Martin Delany had made up his mind that the United States would never accept Blacks as equals or accord them legal rights or even simple justice. "I weary of our miserable condition," he wrote in a letter to the *North Star*, "and am heartily sick of whimpering, whining and snivelling at the feet of the white men, begging for their refuse and offals, existing by mere sufferance."[5]

Delany was choking with rage. The Fugitive Slave Law might have pushed him over the edge, but he, like other free Northern Blacks, had been subjected all his life to racist restrictions that closed off educational possibilities and prohibited civic and professional life. Like all other Black Americans, he lived in an atmosphere heavy with disparagement and opprobrium that marked them as inferior beings.

Delany suffered these conditions, but he rejected them utterly. Growing up free in Pennsylvania, he had been able to go to elementary school. Later several prominent white men had recognized his talent and allowed him to use their libraries, which he did enthusiastically, the start of what became a lifelong habit of reading and learning. He never accepted that he and Blacks in general were naturally inferior in terms of intelligence, energy, or discipline, or in any other way. Psychologically he was endowed with an innate, rock bottom refusal to stomach the derogation. These things had prepared him to be resistant, but they did nothing to quiet his anger.

Together with a group of prominent Black allies, Delany determined to find a way out. In 1852 he wrote and published *The Condition, Elevation, Emigration, and Destiny of the Colored People of the United States*, arguing that because whites would never allow Blacks to coexist as equals, the only solution was "to go from our oppressors." Two years later he convened in Cleveland a National Emigration Convention of Colored People. "No opposition . . . will be entertained," the invitation call announced.[6] Over a hundred delegates attended, discussing, among other topics, the possibilities of Central or South America as potential places for Black resettlement. By the time of the convention, historian Anna Mae Duane writes, "up to 25 percent of the Black population in Ohio favored emigration, a trend echoed by increasing support in Pennsylvania, Maryland, Washington DC, and Vermont."[7] In 1859 Delany undertook a trip to Africa to explore the conditions for establishing a Black American republic in the Yoruba country of the Niger River Valley.

Several pictures of Delany survive. One is a portrait. In it Delany is wearing a US Army uniform, which means it was taken around 1865 when he was about fifty-three years old. He had requested to be assigned as a surgeon to Black Union troops and had been mustered in as a major, the highest ranking Black American to serve in the Civil War. Prior to that he had been granted an interview with President Abraham Lincoln in the White House. There he urged Lincoln to create an army of freed slaves. "I propose, sir," he said to the president, "an army of blacks, commanded by black officers. This army to penetrate the heart of the South, with the banner of Emancipation unfurled, proclaiming freedom as they go. By arming the emancipated, taking them as fresh troops, we would soon have an army of 40,000 blacks in motion It would be an irresistible force."[8] Lincoln sent him to see Secretary of War Edwin Stanton. "Do not fail," Lincoln wrote to Stanton, "to have an interview with this most extraordinary and intelligent black man."[9]

The photograph of Delany is a head-and-shoulder shot. Several rows of large brass buttons show on his uniform. But it's not the buttons that draw attention; it's his face: high forehead, regular features, and a grizzled, close-cut beard. He is a handsome man with a formidable look. But it's his eyes—slightly hooded, intense, intelligent, implacable—that leave an impression.

The emigration controversy persisted until the war, when Emancipation washed over and neutralized it, at least for a time. But until the Battle of Fort Sumter in 1861, emigration was a volatile subject that split the free Black community. It split Delany and Smith's friendship as well. The two men had a great deal in common. They were of an age, born within a year of each other. As abolitionist leaders they wrote and spoke with passion but also with logic and a commanding clarity of thought. Both were close associates of Frederick Douglass. Delany was Douglass's partner in founding *The North Star* and stayed on as coeditor with him for a period of time. Smith wrote a regular column for *The North Star.*

Together with Douglass, he founded the National Council of Colored People, a very early predecessor of the National Association for the Advancement of Colored People (NAACP). Douglass called Smith "the single most important influence on my life" and asked him to write the introduction to his autobiography, *My Bondage and My Freedom*.

Delany's espousal of emigration was a product of disillusion and despair over the possibility of bringing white America to a decent and just accommodation with its Black population. "It is useless to talk about our rights," he wrote in *The Condition, Elevation, Emigration and Destiny of the Colored People*. "We can have no rights here as citizens. . . . Our descent, by the laws of the country, stamps us with inferiority. We are in the hands of the General Government, and no State can rescue us. . . . Heaven and earth— God and Humanity!—are not these sufficient to arouse the most worthless among mankind, of whatever descent, to a sense of their true position?"[10]

Smith thought the opposite. When he returned from his medical studies in Glasgow, he was greeted as a hero by Black New Yorkers. He was an intellectual star, the first university-trained Black physician in America. He had come back to his country— instead of staying in Europe, where a brilliant career awaited him in far more congenial, hate-free surroundings—not just to practice medicine but to fight for his people against slavery and racism. He vowed in front of an enthusiastic lecture-hall crowd "to remain in my native land and to spare no effort and withhold no sacrifice in doing all that I can for the elevation of the American people."[11] He was in for the fight, for his own community, yes, but his community as part of the "American people." An idea like this would have found no place in Delany's Black nationalist frame of reference. "Shake yourself free from these migrating phantasms," Smith wrote. "Our people want to stay, and will stay, at home; we are in for the fight and will fight it out here."

When Smith declared, "We'll fight it out here," he was referring to the ongoing struggle for abolition, equality, and enfranchisement. Legal equality and enfranchisement (for Black men but not for Black women) had to wait three years, until the South was defeated and it was mandated by the Fourteenth Amendment, which passed on July 9, 1868. But it was in the course of the war's bloody progress that the dream of abolition became a reality. Lincoln's Emancipation Proclamation stated that all slaves would be legally free on January 1, 1863, but in fact tens of thousands, and then hundreds of thousands of slaves had already been freeing themselves in the wake of the Union army's progress through Confederate territory.

As the blue armies penetrated farther and farther into the South, slaveowners fled before them, sometimes taking their slaves with them, sometimes just packing whatever they could and abandoning what they couldn't. Often slaves simply emancipated themselves—trickles, then streams, then rivers of refugee men, women, and children attaching themselves to the blue armies. During the Vicksburg campaign in Mississippi, General Ulysses Grant described what was happening in a letter to his sister. "The war is evidently growing oppressive to the Southern people. Their slaves are beginning to have ideas of their own and every time an expedition goes out more or less of them follow in the wake of the army and come into camp."[12] By November 1862 in the Mississippi Valley with its large, lush plantations, 150,000 former slaves were behind Union lines.[13]

In Mississippi and everywhere else the blue armies went, a refugee crisis swelled, overwhelming whatever resources the army could marshal to feed, clothe, and shelter the people who had been freed, or who had freed themselves, but who had left their old homes and way of life with nothing but the clothes on their backs.

Lincoln called them "a laboring, landless, and homeless class," with no plans other than getting away from the places of their enslavement and the potential wrath of their former masters. Many found work with the Union armies as laborers, teamsters, cooks, and launderers. Others joined the ranks of the colored units that began recruiting in the wake of the Emancipation Proclamation. In all, 178,000 Negro solders served during the war's last two years. Many of the colored units were detailed as garrison troops, but others fought in some of the war's fiercest engagements and suffered significantly higher battle deaths than white troops. Twenty-five colored soldiers and sailors received the medal of honor for heroism.

But for most of the emancipated, there were few places to turn. Among the mass of homeless refugees, tens of thousands and ultimately hundreds of thousands drifted into so-called contraband camps that sprung up near army forts and emplacements. In these camps the military attempted to provide some minimal shelter and food. Missionary societies and charitable organizations sent supplies, teachers, nurses, and other aid workers to help educate, organize, and provide the rudiments of desperately needed medical care. But under the best of circumstances, conditions were primitive. More often the camps were squalid, with barely enough to keep people alive and often not even that.

Plantation and farm slaves had always been significantly more vulnerable to disease than the white populations they lived next to. Overall mortality rates and especially infant mortality rates had always been higher, and now the former slaves were further weakened by the physical and emotional stress of flight and wandering, and by living in the crowded, unsanitary conditions of the refugee camps. In the chaos of war and flight, the subsystem of slave health care—the root doctors, midwives, and other healers who attended the health of plantation slaves—dissolved, and the lack of federal preparation meant there was little or nothing to replace them. As one health officer from the 1860s observed, residents existed in "extreme destitution and suffering" with "none of the comforts and few of the necessaries of life."[14]

Medically, the results were disastrous. Two leading historians of African American health, Michael Byrd and Lynda Clayton, conclude, "The end of the Civil War plunged the health of the Black population into what may have been its worst state since the forced African migration to North America."[15] In the postwar years epidemics of the usual killers—smallpox, cholera, and yellow fever—swept through the shattered South, disproportionately affecting the region's destitute Black population. Smallpox targeted Blacks especially. There had been four million slaves, few of whom had ever been inoculated. Throughout the South the Black infant and childhood mortality rate was especially devastating. In Charleston, South Carolina, for example, three times as many Black children under five died as white children in 1868. "It is estimated," historian Herbert Morais writes, "that in some crowded and unhealthy Southern communities from one-quarter to one-third of the former slaves died during the first years of Reconstruction."[16]

During the war, Washington, the country's capital, became a magnet drawing thousands of former slaves toward what they thought would be a haven of safety. As the city filled with newly free men, women, and children—all of them utterly destitute—conditions deteriorated quickly. Contemporary accounts state that public sanitation was almost nonexistent. Pigs, goats, cattle, and chickens roamed freely. "There was an abundance of cheap saloons, gambling houses, low vaudeville houses and other places of cheap entertainment."[17] The refugee influx was so disruptive that the Washington Board of Aldermen delivered a "memorial" to Congress asking it to "provide safeguard against converting the city into an asylum for free Negroes, a population undesirable in any community."[18] To help relieve the situation, the federal government set up employment agencies that found jobs for the refugees, often in far corners of the country. Officials also established camps around the city to house the many thousands who were living in whatever shelter they could find and sustaining themselves however they could.

In 1862 at Camp Barker, one of these local facilities, Congress established the first hospital to provide treatment for the former slave refugees, the so-called Freedmen's Hospital, under the supervision of the Army's Quartermaster Corps. At first Freedmen's Hospital was housed in a couple of old frame buildings that had been set aside to care for the sick and infirm, a gesture toward the idea that the government was responsible for responding to the health needs of the thousands of homeless who were flooding into the city.

In 1865 responsibility for the "hospital" was transferred to the newly established Freedmen's Bureau, which was charged with integrating the former slave population into the general civic life of the country. The Freedmen's Bureau set up schools, food distribution centers, legal aid departments, employment bureaus, and other social welfare programs whose purpose was to cut through the turmoil and toxic racial antipathies faced by the newly emancipated and provide the conditions for self-sustenance, physical safety, and successful entrance into the regular life of the nation.

The man in charge of all this was Oliver Otis Howard, a white Union general who had lost his right arm at the Battle of Seven Pines, a nasty battle that fluctuated back and forth, where he won a medal of honor. Howard, who experienced a religious conversion after graduating from West Point, was known as the "Christian General." The Freedmen's Bureau worked in the South, where enslaved people had lived for generations as illiterate laborers subject to violent often barbaric discipline, whose family lives were unstable at best and in danger of traumatic disruption at the whim of their owners. Integrating four million people who had suffered that level of intellectual, physical, and psychological injury for so long into a population that disdained, maligned, and feared them was an undertaking almost unimaginably immense, a "stupendous work to attempt," W. E. B. Du Bois called it.[19] During the war, Howard had had a mixed record of military success, but he combined in his character the determination, discipline, and utter moral assurance necessary to embrace this daunting mission.

Under the Freedmen's Bureau legislation, Howard wielded wide-ranging power to make decisions regarding all the Southern lands that owners had abandoned or been expelled from during the war, as well as all matters relating to refugees and freedmen from the former rebel states. "Almost unlimited authority," as he described it, "gave me scope and liberty of action."[20] Born in Maine, he had been an ardent abolitionist prior to the war. As the head of this historic agency, he now had the opportunity to give concrete form to his concepts about how to suppress Southern racism and bring about equality for the Negro people.

Among the massive problems Howard took on was the health care of the millions the war had torn loose and abandoned to the elements. Under his lead, the Freedmen's Bureau established more than a hundred hospitals and dispensaries across the South. Freedmen's Hospital in Washington was one of these. Among the hospital's early directors was Alexander T. Augusta, a Black army surgeon who had trained in Canada and had gone to Washington to offer his medical services to the Union army. Augusta continued in the army after the war's conclusion, and then accepted the position at Freedmen's, becoming the first African American to be named a hospital chief administrator.

In 1865 the original ramshackle structures of the hospital were torn down and Freedmen's moved first to temporary buildings, and then to Campbell Hospital, a large facility originally built to take care of wounded soldiers. A year later ground was broken for new construction on land that belonged to what would soon become Howard University.

Howard himself played a central role in founding the university. "The Christian General" was part of Washington's First Congregational Society, which in 1866 decided to establish a school for training African American ministers. During the planning, they expanded their horizons to include teacher training, and that year they founded the Howard Normal and Theological Institute for the Education of Preachers and Teachers. With an eye toward brevity, they soon renamed the school Howard University. Former general Howard had not only a been a driving force in the creation of the university, he had lobbied Congress for formal recognition and had used Freedmen's Bureau money to help pay for the original tract of land.

Howard University was federally chartered in 1867, one of a number of schools of higher learning opened in the South shortly after the war. Howard's attention to Black health care was matched by his feeling about Black education. "The opposition to Negro education made itself felt everywhere," he said,[21] and he was determined to do everything in his power to counter that. Howard University was one effort. He made other personal efforts, including helping found Lincoln Memorial University in eastern Tennessee. The Freedmen's Bureau itself established schools for Blacks and poor whites across the South. Many of the historically Black colleges got their start as part of this postwar movement to address the longing of freed people for education, and the desperate need for it.

Prior to the war the abolitionist movement had given birth to a very few, lonely institutions of higher learning for Blacks. Cheney State College in Pennsylvania was the first, founded by Quakers in 1837 to provide agricultural, mechanical, and teacher training. Lincoln University (originally Ashmun Institute), also in Pennsylvania, came second in 1854. Two years later Wilberforce University was founded in Ohio by the African Methodist Episcopal (AME) Church in conjunction with the Ohio Conference of the white Methodist Episcopal Church, but after the war the AME Church assumed sole ownership, making Wilberforce University the first Black-owned and -administered college in the country. In 1863 the physician, scholar, abolitionist, and prominent member of the country's Black intelligentsia James McCune Smith, Martin Delany's old adversary, was appointed professor of anthropology there; unfortunately, by that time he was too ill with congestive heart failure to assume the position.

More than a few of the postwar institutions had relatively brief lives, but others survived, at times going through name changes, mergers, and later affiliations with state educational systems. Some of those early schools are well-known historically Black colleges and universities today—Atlanta (now Atlanta Clark) University, Dillard University, Fisk University, Alcorn State University, Morehouse College, and Tougaloo College, among others. But Howard University stands out for establishing the first medical department, in 1867. The following year, Freedmen's Hospital became Howard's teaching hospital.

Physicians of that period, looking for advancement in the profession, applied for membership in their local medical society; in Washington that was the Medical Society of the District of Columbia (MSDC). In June 1869 two African American faculty members in Howard's medical department—Drs. Alexander Augusta and Charles Purvis—applied for membership. Both had been Union army surgeons. They were joined by a third African American doctor, Alpheus Tucker. All were reported as qualified for admission. All were rejected.[22]

Ironically, this took place at the exact moment Congress was debating the proposed Fourteenth Amendment to the Constitution guaranteeing equal rights. Massachusetts Senator Charles Sumner, a militant advocate for Black equality, went to the floor of the Senate to remonstrate: "Thus do members of the society constitute themselves as a medical oligarchy. . . . [T]hese white oligarchs ought to have notice, and I give them notice now that this outrage shall not be allowed to continue. . . . [T]he time has passed for any such pretention."[23]

The Society responded, saying that membership was not a professional matter but a personal and social one. Sumner then submitted a bill to repeal the Society's charter. If the Medical Society of the District of Columbia wasn't a professional organization, but just a social club, then it was simply "a nuisance and a shame."[24] The Senate declined to act on the bill.

Over the next eight months, the African American physicians applied again for membership with the support of Dr. Robert Reyburn, a white professor at Howard and chief surgeon at the Freedmen's Hospital. Their second set of applications received the same treatment as their first. That wasn't the end of the fight, though. Rebuffed by the Medical Society of the District of Columbia, Howard's integrated medical department took the conflict to the next level. At a meeting in January 1870, some of the members decided to form an alternative medical society whose membership would be open to all. This they did, founding the integrated *National Medical Society* of the District of Columbia. The new society then sent a memorial to Congress protesting the actions of the old society: "It is a fact worthy of note, that this is the only country and the only profession in which such a distinction [of color] is made. Science knows no race, color, or condition, and we protest against the Medical Society of the District of Columbia maintaining such a relic of barbarism."[25]

Matters came to a head at the May 1870 National Convention of the American Medical Association, the umbrella organization for all state and local societies. Here, both Washington, DC, societies—the all-white MSDC and the integrated National Medical Society (NMS)—submitted applications for members to be seated as delegates. The all-white Society argued that members of the integrated society not be seated as delegates because it had instigated a congressional investigation of the MSDC, which threatened their authorization by the American Medical Association (AMA)—they were referring to Senator Sumner's bill, which had been "passed over" in committee, that is, not voted on. The NMS argued back, accusing the MSDC of racial discrimination. When the roll call of accredited members was read off on the first day of the convention, all the MSDC members were seated, and none of the NMS society were.

With business underway, the matter was referred to the AMA's Ethics Committee for resolution. On the second day, another white Howard faculty member, Dr. Silas Loomis, entered a motion to admit all the Washington, DC, candidates pending the Ethics Committee report. Loomis's motion was defeated 142 to 107.

The Ethics Committee reported its findings on the convention's next to last day. There was a minority report and a majority report. The minority report recommended the inclusion of the NMS members, declaring the NMS was "regularly organized," the excluded physicians were qualified practitioners of medicine, and there were "no sufficient grounds" for exclusion. The majority report recommended excluding NMS members because the NMS had "used unfair and dishonorable means" to procure the destruction of the

MSDC and because some of the NMS members were not licensed.[26] (Licenses in Washington, DC, were issued by the MSDC, which had started the entire battle by refusing to accept Black members.)

The majority report was adopted by a vote of 114 to 82. The minority report was tabled by a vote of 112 to 80. A second vote was called on a motion by Dr. John L. Sullivan from Massachusetts: "Resolved, That no distinction of race or color shall exclude from the Association persons claiming admission and duly accredited thereto." This motion was tabled by a vote of 106 to 60.

It's notable that the majority report of the AMA Ethics Committee was authored by Dr. Nathan Smith Davis, often called the father of the AMA. A leader in the push for national medical education requirements, Davis voted with the Southerners on the Ethics Committee, although he himself was born and raised in New York and achieved prominence in Chicago as the founder of what became the Northwestern University School of Medicine. His appeasement of the racist Southern medical establishment was likely born of a conviction that keeping the South within the national medical standards movement overrode the moral principle of recognizing the equality of all qualified physicians. His complicity was a key element in the AMA's decision that it would do nothing to prevent local or state medical societies from excluding African American physicians from membership. The result was that Southern, border state, and many Northern medical societies did exclude Black applicants, who were thus excluded from the AMA.

For medicine, the consequences were profound—the decision was self-destructive for American health care in general, and was devastating for Black physicians and thus for all African Americans. Many states required membership in the state medical society as a prerequisite for admitting patients to hospitals, which meant that Black physicians were denied hospital privileges. Being shut out of medical societies commonly meant that white physicians refused to consult with their Black peers, and restricted access to professional training and continuing medical education. Black doctors had nowhere to turn to improve their professional standing, acquire additional skills and knowledge, and provide comprehensive care for their patients. AMA exclusion was a key factor in creating the two-tiered health care system that bears a large responsibility for the pronounced health care inequities that African Americans still suffer from in 2021.

The AMA's exclusionary policies lasted well into the twentieth century. It wasn't until 1968—almost a hundred years after the infamous 1870 convention—that the AMA changed its bylaws to prohibit segregation in local societies. It took an additional forty years for the AMA to issue a formal apology for segregation. That initial post–Civil War rejection of Black equality by the nation's medical establishment led to an era that is sometimes referred to as "The Nadir" in African American health care. It was a time when Black society was thrown onto its own scant resources as it struggled to care for its own.

CHAPTER 2

The Response

"The ravages of disease are increasing with a fearful ratio among the colored people. . . . We see the problem of the negro's [*sic*] future dark with gloom." That was the opinion of the president of the Memphis Board of Health in 1887.[1] The insurance industry outlook for America's Black population was similarly bleak; by 1881 major companies essentially stopped writing life insurance for African Americans. The reason they gave was the elevated mortality rates.[2]

Post–Civil War morbidity and mortality numbers indicate that they had a point. In five large Southern and border cities (Louisville, Baltimore, New Orleans, St. Louis, and Washington, DC), the 1880 census reported that the death rate for white children under five was 88.48 per thousand; for "colored" it was 151.60.[3] In New Orleans in 1880, of one thousand Black infants born, some 450 died.[4] Life expectancy for Black males in 1900 was about thirty-five years.[5] In the 1890s the Black child mortality rate was 50 percent above the white rate.[6] African Americans living in cities tended to concentrate in the poorest, most congested neighborhoods, with no sanitation, unhealthy drinking water, and little access to adequate nutrition. The health statistics reflected the circumstances, with tuberculosis, a disease associated with poverty, being the major killer.

In the rural South, home to almost 90 percent of the African American population, health care most often simply did not exist. In Georgia, for example, in 1890 there was one Black physician for every 21,470 African Americans.[7] With no African American doctors available, with only the rare Black hospital, and with no transportation, most rural Blacks had no health care other than the traditional remedies. When Louis Sullivan, one of this book's authors, was growing up in the south Georgia town of Blakely in the 1930s, the health care situation had not changed since post–Civil War times. There was one Black doctor in the area, whose clinic was forty miles away. Sullivan's father, a mortician, had one of the very few Black-owned cars, a hearse. If someone was sick enough to go to the doctor, he would transport them. "In later years," Sullivan said, "I used to think how those patients must have felt— sick enough to make the long trip to Dr. Griffin, and picked up for that trip by the undertaker in his hearse."

Future surgeon general Joycelyn Elders, growing up at the same time in a sharecropper family in rural Arkansas, never considered the possibility of seeing a doctor. If someone was sick or injured,

> you were on your own. You weren't going to go up to the hospital emergency room and get it fixed. There wasn't any hospital. You weren't going to make an appointment to see your family doctor. You didn't have a doctor. If Chester [Elders's brother] stepped on a nail, you put coal oil on it and prayed that this wasn't the nail that was going to give him lockjaw. If Pat [Elders's sister] was attacked by a strange dog, you waited to see if that dog had rabies in its bite. And your anxiety level shot right up. You weren't calm. Because you

knew people who had died grinning with tetanus or deranged with hydrophobia.[8]

Sullivan and Elders were born more than fifty years after the 1880 census, which recorded such appalling Black morbidity and mortality statistics. It's little wonder that by the time of the 1890 census, many politicians, physicians, and even Frederick Hoffman, the chief statistician of the Prudential Insurance Company, were predicting the eventual demise of the African American population. Although Hoffman was a leading statistician of the period, he was also a racist who failed to take into account any of the environmental factors that so significantly weighted the Black mortality numbers. Other racist factors contributed to the extinction projection, including prevailing ideas about Black physiological inferiority and inherent Black vulnerability to various diseases. The idea that the Black population might actually die off was comprised of improbabilities and racist assumptions—it was a myth. But myth or not, the possibility was a part of the national conversation.

In this environment of health care deprivation and the medical establishment's hostility to Black physicians, the African American community and its white allies began generating a response, and Howard University's medical department and the Freedmen's Hospital were the start. These two institutions were key in developing the federal government's awareness that it had some level of responsibility for the care of the former slaves—a "revolutionary development," as one leading historian put it, the first instance of Washington's assumption of health care responsibility for the poor and indigent. The hospital was a Freedmen's Bureau undertaking, as was Howard and its medical school; funding from the Bureau had enabled the school to buy land and construct its early buildings. But the Freedmen's Bureau itself was closed down in 1872. The seven years of its existence marked the heart of Reconstruction, and when it shut its doors, the lifeline of funding for the schools and hospitals the Bureau had established withered and died, including the funding for Howard University. Fortunately, in 1879, the school prevailed on Congress to provide an annual subsidy, which Howard still receives today.

Located in the nation's capital, Howard had an ongoing government affiliation, as well as close connections to Washington's liberal elite. It was open to all—the medical school's entering class included a white male student, along with seven African Americans (the university's entering class included five white women). During the medical school's early period, most of its students were from the North. Others came from the West Indies and even foreign countries. The Howard medical school was diverse and cosmopolitan, practically from the outset.[9]

Howard's graduates constituted the first flow of African American physicians into the American health care scene. It was a phenomenon then, and the emergence of minority physicians and their integration into the world of health professionals is still, a hundred and fifty years later, a charged subject in terms of unequal access and insufficient numbers.[10] Howard's graduate doctors in the postbellum world were well-trained, but the numbers were sparse, particularly given the immensity of the need. From 1871 through 1890, Howard graduated 238 male physicians and fourteen female physicians,[11] many of whom came from the North and went back home to open practices. As a result, their impact on the health of the vast former slave population was not substantial.

Reconstruction opened up educational opportunities for a people who had been utterly deprived and who possessed a deep well of desire to acquire not simply the essential tools of literacy and numeracy but a higher level of skills and knowledge. The Freedmen's Bureau had established schools throughout the South—elementary, secondary, and some higher-level institutions. Nongovernmental aid organizations also threw themselves into the endeavor, in particular the American Missionary Association and its Freedmen's Aid Society, composed of Congregationalists, Methodists, Presbyterians, and members of other church communions committed to abolition first, then education and integration. From the beginning the Missionary Association's leadership included African Americans who dedicated themselves to helping their own suppressed brothers and sisters. During the war the Association sent nurses and teachers into the contraband camps. Afterward the organization established schools and colleges throughout the former Confederacy.

One of these was Central Tennessee College in Nashville, founded first as a community school, then expanded. In 1866 the Freedmen's Bureau funneled money into the construction of the school's first buildings. A decade later Central Tennessee added the Meharry Medical Department, named for the five white Meharry brothers who provided a major part of the initial funding.

The origin of this funding is part of Meharry Medical College's foundation story, and is not widely known outside of Meharry circles. The story, passed down years later by Samuel Meharry, is that in the 1820s, Meharry, as a sixteen-year-old, was hauling a load of salt in Tennessee when his wagon slid into a muddy rut. Unable to extricate it, and with night and rain coming on, the young Samuel went searching for help and came across a cabin that was home to a family of freed slaves. The family offered him shelter and food and the next morning helped him get the wagon back on the road. The family's helpfulness was as courageous as it was kind. Interactions with strange white people put manumitted slaves at risk of reenslavement.[12] According to the story, Samuel told them that he had no money but that when he did, he would find a way to repay their kindness (in the handed-down story, he said, "I shall do something for your race"). Many years later,

Samuel Meharry learned about Central Tennessee College's desire to establish a medical department. Prosperous by then, he repaid the debt by contributing funds, bringing his four brothers with him as codonors.

From the start, Meharry was different from Howard. During the war, the school's (white) founding president, George Whipple Hubbard, had served as an assistant chaplain with Sherman's army. In the war's last year, he was assigned to teach troops of the Tenth Colored Infantry stationed in Tennessee, and when the war was over, he was appointed principal of the Belleview School, one of the public schools established by the Nashville Board of Education for the instruction "of the colored scholastic population."[13] For seven years Hubbard oversaw the education of Negro youngsters before he enrolled at Vanderbilt's medical college, where he earned a medical degree in 1876. That same year, the American Missionary Association asked Hubbard to help establish a medical department at Central Tennessee College.

Hubbard was then thirty-five years old. He had spent a good deal of his adult life in the South teaching Black students. Both he and the Missionary Association were dedicated to providing education for the South's African American population, and his medical training pointed him toward the vast deficit in health care. At Central Tennessee he was joined by Dr. William Sneed, who had served as a surgeon with the Confederate Army, then as a professor at Vanderbilt (then Nashville) School of Medicine when Hubbard was a student there. Together the two men—Hubbard, the inveterate educator, and Sneed, an accomplished clinician and academic—brought their talents and drive to plan Central Tennessee's medical department, which was given the resources by the Meharry brothers.

Unlike Howard, Meharry was, from the start, a Southern school dedicated to the medical education of African American students, specifically to serve in the health care desert of the former slave states. While most of Howard's medical enrollees came with a standard educational background, that wasn't true of Meharry, which drew its students from the poor South. Some were former slaves, some the children of former slaves, and typically had to work any kind of job they could get to support themselves while they were studying. Often they needed substantial remedial work before they were ready for the medical curriculum. That was reflected in the graduation rates during the first few years. Meharry's entering medical class included eleven students. Of these, only one graduated in the first year of eligibility; three graduated the following year.

Between 1877 and 1890, Meharry graduated 102 students as physicians, most of them opening practices in the South. "From its origins," historians Byrd and Clayton write, "Meharry Medical College was organic to the Black community."[14] The small number of graduates grew substantially, and the school's impact grew accordingly, furnishing dozens and then many hundreds of grassroots family physicians for a people who had had little or no access to health care previously.

Both Howard and Meharry early on recognized the parallel need for African American dentists as well as doctors, and both established dental schools in the 1880s. African American doctors, from their earliest emergence, had practiced dentistry, or at least tooth extraction, along with medicine. Among others, John Swett Rock was a mid-nineteenth-century physician and dentist. Like his contemporaries Martin Delany and James McCune Smith, Rock was a militant abolitionist who combined his medical and dental practice with relentless anti-slavery activism. (Later in his life, when illness forced Rock to give up his medical and dental practice, he began to study law. He soon developed a successful legal career in Boston and in 1865 became the first Black to be admitted to practice before the Supreme Court.)

Later in the century, Dr. Robert Boyd received both an MD and DDS from Meharry and worked as a physician and dentist, building a major practice in Nashville and prominence as a professor of gynecology and clinical medicine at Meharry. Boyd, like Rock, was one of the leading Black physicians of his day. Both of these accomplished men became dentists at least in part because, given the many racial barriers Black physicians faced, building a financially successful medical practice was far from assured. "Double degrees were not uncommon at this time," physician and anthropologist Montague Cobb wrote in the *Journal of the National Medical Association* in 1953. "In those days the practice of medicine was considered a very doubtful means of livelihood for a colored man. Dr. Boyd was the first Negro to make that venture in Nashville."[15]

The same need to double-up on professions prevailed in Washington, DC, among Howard medical graduates, who then went on to get dentistry degrees. Howard also opened a pharmacy department, first as part of the medical curriculum, then as a separate program. Many African American graduates who earned an MD also earned a pharmacy degree there. Like dentistry, pharmacy had a history among Black healers. Given the plant expertise of traditional practitioners, pharmacy was, in a sense, a natural vocation. The eighteenth-century doctor Primus Manumit spent the years of his apprenticeship compounding medicines, as did other apprentice-trained Black doctors. In New York James McCune Smith established what was probably the country's first Black-owned pharmacy at 93 West Broadway in present-day Tribeca. With Howard and Meharry as forerunners, the twentieth century saw the rise of other Black dental and pharmacy schools: Xavier University, Hampton University, Florida A&M University, and Texas Southern University.

Meharry and Howard transformed the landscape of Black medicine. But even together, the two schools couldn't begin to satisfy the demand for African American health practitioners. From established white medical schools there was no help. None of the Southern or border state schools would accept Black applicants. A few Northern schools did, but only in token numbers. In the high-demand Southern environment, additional Black medical schools opened their doors; some were started by missionary societies, others were proprietary, founded by enterprising Black physicians. The largest of these was Leonard Medical School at Shaw University in Raleigh, North Carolina, sponsored by the American Baptist Home Missionary Society. Others included Straight University Medical Department and Flint Medical College, both located in New Orleans, and Louisville National Medical College. All were fragile financially, although those with church or university backing were slightly less precarious. The proprietary schools were often funded out of their founders' pockets and had no resources to speak of to accommodate the increasingly stringent demands of up-to-date medical education. As a result, although the post–Howard and Meharry schools expanded the flow of trained African American physicians, few schools enjoyed any significant longevity. Howard and Meharry were the only two to survive the hard assessments of the 1910 Flexner Report, by educator and reformer Abraham Flexner, who evaluated all the medical schools in the country based on their method of teaching and their graduation standards. Flexner determined which American medical schools had the ability to restructure themselves according to the new biomedical model represented by the Johns Hopkins School of Medicine.

~

The post–Civil War chaos of several million newly homeless former slaves, a massive refugee movement, and an inadequate government response that had to be built from scratch—all in a setting of racial antipathy—generated a shock wave felt in every dimension of American life. For African Americans, the hard reality of Emancipation manifested in part as morbidity and mortality—that is, disease and death. In response, the Black community, with help from its white allies, began forging a health care structure to serve its own needs. Medical, pharmacy, and dental schools made their appearance. In the face of segregation and exclusion, so did hospitals and nursing schools.

The first Black nursing school, combined with a hospital, was willed into existence by Daniel Hale Williams, one of several African American graduates of the Chicago Medical College. In 1883 Williams opened a practice in Chicago, the third Black doctor in the city to do so, but he was unable to acquire hospital privileges at any of Chicago's established hospitals, despite his developing reputation as a skilled surgeon. (Ten years later Williams performed one of the first open heart surgeries, a successful suturing of the pericardial sac of a man who had been stabbed in the chest.) African American practitioners of that era were effectively shut out of hospital affiliations, which drastically limited their ability to take full care of their patients and advance their own skills.

In 1890 the pastor of Williams's AME church asked him to help place a young African American woman who had been rejected by Chicago's nursing schools because of her race. Something about this young woman's plight pushed Williams over the line. Known for his single-minded dedication to his work as a physician and surgeon, Williams turned activist. This particular young woman was not alone. Chicago nursing schools would not accept any Black candidates for admission. The answer to this particular injustice, Williams thought, is to establish a nursing school for African American students as well as a hospital for them to train in.

Williams first consulted with the few other Black doctors in Chicago and with a group of Black ministers and businessmen. When their responses were enthusiastic, he began to raise support among Black community members, who were equally encouraging. At the same time, he also raised funds among Chicago's wealthy elite, including George Pullman, Cyrus McCormick, the meat-packing Armour family, and retailing and real estate mogul Palmer Potter.

With donations from the wealthy and from Chicago's Black community, in 1891 Williams opened the twelve-bed Provident Hospital. "The object for which it is formed," the charter declared, "is to maintain a hospital and training school for nurses in the city of Chicago, Illinois, for the gratuitous treatment of the medical and surgical diseases of the sick poor." A building campaign six years later enabled the hospital to move to larger quarters. With Williams as chief of staff, Provident Hospital's patients were both Black and white, as were its attending physicians. Colored nurses now had a place to train, and colored physicians had an institution that would grant them hospital experience and privileges.

With the opening of Provident Hospital, Williams led the way in what became known as the Black Hospital Movement. Provident Hospital was followed by others—Tuskegee Institute Hospital and Nurse Training School in 1892, Provident Hospital in Baltimore in 1894, and Frederick Douglass Memorial Hospital and Training School in Philadelphia in 1895, which was founded by Nathan Francis Mossell, the first Black graduate of the University of Pennsylvania Medical School, the oldest medical school in the country. Mossell, like Williams, was undaunted by racist hostility. He had applied for admission directly to Pennsylvania's dean, Dr. James Tyson. Tyson was impressed. At the interview's end he told Mossell, "We have a greater medical school than Harvard or Yale, and since they have admitted Negroes, we will."[16]

Before the opening lecture of the 1879 term, Mossell was told he'd have to sit behind a screen. He refused to do that. Instead, he walked down the middle aisle of the amphitheater and took a seat in front, which occasioned a storm of protest and cries of "Put the nigger out!" Recalling the event later, he wrote, "A student by whom I sat asked me why I did not get up and tell them, 'go to hell.' I replied that I was not disturbed the least bit; whereupon he jumped on the seat, turned his face to the crowd, and said in a ringing voice, 'Go to hell! You act like a pack of D__ fools.' In response he got some applause, making me know that everyone had not participated in the first demonstration."[17]

After Mossell received his degree from Penn, he trained with the medical school's distinguished professor of surgery David Hays Agnew. (A famous painting by Thomas Eakins portrays Agnew performing a mastectomy in Penn's operating theater.) Subsequently he spent a number of years in London at Guys, Queens, and St. Thomas Hospitals, where he met Black American students and Black professors. Regarding English institutions, he wrote: "Where education and job promotions are concerned . . . prejudice against people of color is an unknown entity."[18]

Philadelphia was a very different story; aspiring Black physicians and nurses were unable to find institutions there open to them. "Caste prejudice," Mossell wrote, "in the hearts of the dominant race, in charge of the numerous hospitals and training schools in our city made it impossible for the capable and ambitious colored nurses and physicians to secure hospital experience."[19] In Chicago Daniel Williams had been driven by the city's need for a hospital that would care for the "sick poor" and provide training for Black nurses and physicians. In Philadelphia Mossell was driven by the same conviction, which led to the founding of the Frederick Douglas Memorial Hospital and Training School, where he served as chief of staff for the next thirty-five years.

Chicago, Tuskegee, Baltimore, and Philadelphia were homes to the first interracial hospitals after Freedmen's. They were the spearhead of a movement to establish hospitals that would serve

Black patients. By 1900 there were some forty of these around the country, which made hospital care available to African Americans, at least those who lived near enough to access them. These hospitals provided nursing training and also gave Black physicians hospital affiliations, which were closed to them in the segregated white hospitals.

Together with Howard and Meharry, and the other Black medical schools that came into being in the late nineteenth century, these hospitals and training schools constituted a response to the catastrophic health situation of the country's postwar African American population during "the worst state since the forced African migration to North America," as Byrd and Clayton have written.[20] In the most desperate part of that "forced migration," newly enslaved Africans on those Middle Passage ships had demonstrated their determination to fight against the circumstances they found themselves in and to establish connection and mutual support in the face of their oppressors. Those same instincts were still alive and well as the now-emancipated community struggled to respond to the bleakness of its new situation.

The heroism of men like Daniel Hale Williams and Nathan Francis Mossell was a complex of toughness, drive, moral sense, and a profound identification with and compassion for their fellow African Americans. The depth of the skepticism and hostility they faced can be judged from the Pennsylvania Medical School faculty's explanation to Mossell after they voted to admit him; he was "an experiment," they told him, and they couldn't be responsible "if anything happened to him." The school's trustees wondered if "the Negro mind [would] be able to comprehend higher education."[21]

Even after his graduation and surgical training with David Hays Agnew, that same ingrained racist psychology raised its head again when Mossell applied for membership in the Philadelphia Medi-

tion had hardly dissipated, but by the 1880s and '90s, a pragmatic sense had taken hold. In order to move forward, Black physicians needed to look to themselves. The hospitals were one element, as were the medical schools and nursing institutions, the pharmacy and dental schools, and now the medical societies, which spoke to the need for connection among the growing number of Black doctors and other health care professionals.

The men who established the first Black medical societies understood the benefits, and the necessity, of organization and connection. Dr. Myles Vandarhurst Lynk took that understanding to the next level. Dr. Lynk had been a precocious child. He had supplemented his limited rural school education with intensive, curiosity-driven reading in history, biography, current events, and other subjects. He was, he said, "a graduate of Pine Knot College."[25] At the age of thirteen he passed the exam for a teaching certificate in his home state of Tennessee—which he couldn't use because of his youth. At nineteen he graduated second in his class from Meharry. Two years later, in 1892, he founded the first national medical journal for Black doctors, dentists, and pharmacists, *The Medical and Surgical Observer*. *The Observer* was a platform for sharing medical information especially among the almost four hundred Black doctors then practicing in many parts of the country, often in isolated settings. Lynk also used the journal to call for a national association of African American physicians.

That idea percolated for several years until in 1895 Lynk visited the Cotton States and International Exposition in Atlanta. Meharry's Robert Boyd was also visiting the exposition, as was Daniel Hale Williams from Chicago. When the three of them met, they discussed, among other things, the idea of a national organization. It seemed to these three powerhouses of Black medicine that not only was the time ripe but also it didn't make sense to waste any more of it. By the next day they had spoken with the nine or ten other Black doctors in attendance and had asked Garland Penn, who had organized the Black exhibits at the exposition, to chair a meeting.

When Penn asked the doctors for their thoughts on starting such an organization, the sense was that the need was palpable. The doctors voted to move ahead, and then they elected Boyd president and Williams vice president. They named the organization the Society of Colored Physicians and Surgeons, which was later changed to the National Medical Association.

Looking back on that founding moment, the fifth president of the Association, Dr. Charles Roman, defined the meaning the organization had for its founders: "Conceived in no spirit of racial exclusiveness, fostering no ethnic antagonisms, but born of the exigencies of the American environment, the National Medical Association has for its object the banding together for mutual cooperation and helpfulness, the men and women of African descent who are legally and honorably engaged in the practice of the cognate professions of medicine, surgery, pharmacy and dentistry."[26]

The NMA's establishment was a watershed in the centuries-long story of Black medicine and health care in America. It's a story that moves through stages: the traditional healers who brought African practices with them to the American plantations; the interaction with white American doctoring; the emergence into the mainstream of the first few Black physicians; the rise of Black medical institutions and the early flow from their doors of graduates who were educated as doctors, dentists, pharmacists and nurses; the banding together for mutual aid of African American doctors in their own societies; and now, nearly three hundred years after Africans first arrived in the American colonies, a nationwide mobilization of Black physicians. In 1860 James McCune Smith had declared in his opposition to emigration, "We are in for the fight, and we will fight it out here." With the National Medical Association, African American physicians for the first time were positioned, as Byrd and Clayton put it, "to take on the struggle of Black people in America for justice and equity in healthcare."[27]

CHAPTER 3

Abraham Flexner and the Black Medical Schools

Robert Fulton Boyd, the National Medical Association's first president, was born into plantation slavery in Tennessee in either 1855 or 1858. His childhood was spent as a field hand. Some sources say that when he was eight, his mother brought him to Nashville to live with the family of Dr. Paul Eve, a renowned white surgeon who was a professor at Vanderbilt School of Medicine. It isn't known what the connection between Boyd's family and Eve might have been, although it's possible that the plantation where Boyd was born was owned by the Eve family. In Nashville, Boyd worked and attended night school, then entered Fisk School (later Fisk University) where he learned to read and write, although when he was thirteen, as he recounted later, he still "knew but the elements of reading."[1]

But at Fisk School he did learn, and in 1880, after stints as a bricklayer and teacher, he entered Meharry Medical College, graduating with an MD two years later. But it wasn't until he earned a further degree in dentistry at Meharry that he opened a medical practice and finally launched himself on what became a distinguished medical career. The National Medical Association, which Boyd presided over for three years, was at first only a name rather than a functioning organization. Given the exclusion and isolation of most of the country's four hundred or so Black physicians (Boyd was the first Black doctor to establish a practice in Nashville), it is surprising that the association survived at all. The NMA's founding gathering was in 1895, but there is no record of further meetings until 1898. Boyd, Daniel Hale Williams, Myles Lynk, and the other nine Black physicians who founded the NMA at Atlanta's Cotton States Exhibit envisioned an association that could eventually serve Black health professionals as a counterpart to the whites-only American Medical Association.

But the effort to build membership and mobilize support to address the profound health deficits suffered by African Americans turned out to be a long, slow slog. It took another ten years for the NMA to become a force in Black medicine and eventually an important player on the national health scene. Boyd himself developed a thriving medical and dental practice in Nashville and was appointed professor of anatomy and physiology at Meharry Medical College. After attending courses at the Chicago Post-Graduate School of Medicine in surgery and women's health and doing clinical work at various Chicago hospitals, he returned to Meharry to head the school's departments of gynecology and clinical medicine. With his experience in Chicago as background, in 1890 Boyd founded the twenty-three-bed Mercy Hospital in Nashville, which became Meharry's teaching hospital.

In Chicago, Boyd had studied and worked under the supervision of some of the country's most accomplished clinicians. In his own practice in Nashville, he was renowned not just for his skill but for his care and determination with both white and Black patients, and for the special attention he gave to the poor. It's not too much to say that he was widely regarded as the foremost Black physician of his day.

If Boyd was the leading Black American physician, a contemporary of his from Connecticut, William Welch, was to become the most influential white physician, whose work did much to determine the future course of American medicine. Welch, like Boyd, was driven throughout his life to constantly increase his understanding of disease and treatment. Like Boyd, Welch founded a hospital. But their differences illustrate the vast gulf between white and Black medicine and health care that forged the two-tiered system that has been so detrimental to Black health, the residual effects of which have reached well into the twenty-first century.

While Boyd was born into slavery, William Henry Welch was born into a family rich with physicians and surgeons. His grandfather, his father, and two of his uncles practiced medicine. According to Welch's eulogist, Harvey Cushing, himself a famous surgeon, "There must have been at least ten doctors in three generations [of the Welch family]."[2] While Boyd was struggling to learn his three *R*s at night school and part-time while he worked, Welch attended private schools, then enrolled at Yale in 1866 at the age of sixteen. At Yale he studied the classics. After flirting with the idea of teaching Greek and Latin, he went on to study medicine at the Columbia University College of Physicians and Surgeons.

In the late nineteenth century, medical science was expanding the understanding of disease at a dizzying pace. But American medical schools like Columbia were far behind in their engagement with the biomedical dimension of disease. The College of Physicians and Surgeons, for example, had no scientific laboratories when Welch was a student there. "American medical schools contributed virtually nothing to medical science in the second half of the 19th century," according to medical historian John Duffy.

"American medical graduates who wished to keep up with the latest in medicine were forced to study abroad."[3]

In terms of medical science, Germany was the acknowledged leader. Rudolf Virchow, thought by many to be the foremost medical scientist in history, taught and ran laboratories at the Friedrich Wilhelm University in Berlin and at the University of Würzburg, where he was appointed to Germany's first chair in pathological anatomy. Virchow originated and pioneered the cell theory of disease, among other breakthroughs in the understanding of disease origin, and many of his students became leading medical scientists in their own right. Once Welch completed his studies at Columbia, he left for Germany in order to study in Strasbourg and then Leipzig with several of Virchow's most prominent proteges.

The late nineteenth century was an extraordinary time not just for specific medical breakthroughs but for a fundamental transformation of medicine and surgery. The etiology of disease had been the great mystery of health and health care throughout the ages. By the middle of the nineteenth century, the ancient concept of *humors* still prevailed, the idea that disease was caused by imbalances in what was believed to be the four constituent elements of human physiology and temperament: blood, black and yellow bile, and phlegm. The idea of humors was complemented by and eventually overtaken by *miasma* theory—the belief that the great killer diseases, like yellow fever, cholera, tuberculosis, and malaria, were caused by inhaling poisonous emanations from the environment: rotting organic elements, swamps, bad atmospheric conditions, and so on. Benjamin Rush believed, for example, that the great 1793 yellow fever epidemic in Philadelphia was caused by foul emanations from a large shipment of coffee that had been left to rot on the city's docks. His treatment for the disease consisted of repeated bloodlettings and heroic doses of cathartics to right the resulting imbalances.

But during the latter half of the nineteenth century, the discovery of bacteria by Leeuwenhoek, the seminal advances in germ
theory by Pasteur, and the discoveries and evolving understanding of cell biology by Virchow and others led to a thoroughgoing
transformation of the medical establishment's understanding of
disease and its origins. In a relatively short period, science replaced
speculation with *knowledge* when determining disease origin, which
enabled revolutionary advances in therapeutics, vaccination, surgery, and obstetrics. Immunology research flourished, resulting in
the development of vaccines for anthrax, rabies, typhoid fever,
cholera, and bubonic plague. Karl Landsteiner's discovery of blood
types allowed for safe transfusions, and Wilhelm Roentgen's work
with X-rays gave birth to radiological diagnoses.

The world of modern medical science was born largely in Europe in the last decades of the nineteenth century, but was only
slowly appreciated in American medical schools. "I was often
asked in Germany," Welch wrote, "how it is that no scientific work
in medicine is done in this country, how it is that many good men
who do well in Germany and show evident talent there are never
heard of and never do any good work when they come back here.
The answer is that there is no opportunity for, no appreciation of,
no demand for that kind of work here. In Germany on the other
hand every encouragement is held out for young men with a taste
for science."[4]

Welch was eager to change that. When he returned to the
United States in 1877, he first proposed to introduce laboratory science at Columbia's School of Physicians and Surgeons but was met
with a chilly lack of enthusiasm. He had better luck at Bellevue,
where he was given a couple of unused rooms but no money for
equipment and no salary, which meant he had to open a private
practice to sustain himself. Then, in 1884 he got the chance of a

lifetime when he was interviewed for the position of professor at the newly conceived Johns Hopkins School of Medicine.

Johns Hopkins was a radical departure in medical education, "the most spectacular innovation in the history of American medical education," writes historian Kenneth Ludmerer, although Ludmerer also notes that reforms at Harvard, the University of Michigan, and the University of Pennsylvania predated the opening of Johns Hopkins.[5] While the course of study at most American schools was two or three years, Johns Hopkins initiated a four-year curriculum, where the first two years were devoted to the basic sciences that undergirded the new understanding of disease. Sociologist Paul Starr writes, "From the outset, Johns Hopkins embodied a conception of medical education . . . rooted in basic science and hospital medicine that was eventually to govern all institutions in the country. Scientific research and clinical instruction now moved to center stage."[6] Applicants to the school were carefully selected, and a bachelor's degree was required as a prerequisite for admission since only well-prepared students would be capable of absorbing the new knowledge—this at a time when a great many medical school applicants were barely literate.

Welch was Johns Hopkins School of Medicine's first professor and founding dean. In short order he helped recruit three other "founding professors" who were preeminent in their own specialties: William Osler in clinical medicine, Stewart Halsted in surgery, and Howard Kelly in gynecology. Whereas most medical schools relied on local doctors to staff their faculties, each of the original professors at Johns Hopkins was a clinician/scientist of national stature.

⁓

The innovations at Johns Hopkins set new standards for American schools of medicine that raised the level of American medical education in unprecedented ways. The new model programs and schools were also, not incidentally, so expensive that they up-ended the traditional financial model of medical schools, which had always relied on student tuitions to pay teachers and main-tain physical plants. Biomedical science-based schools required modern laboratories, specialized research equipment, trained technicians, extensive medical libraries, and research faculty who were not overburdened by teaching duties and did not have energy-absorbing private practices that gave them income but di-verted them from scientific investigation.

Exploding costs required large gifts and endowment funding, along with higher fees from students and patients in affiliated teaching hospitals. Schools without access to new sources of in-come had no ability to upgrade themselves to the emerging stan-dards. This was true for many of the 148 medical schools in the country, including the fourteen Black schools that had established themselves in the post–Civil War years, seven of which were still functioning when William Welch was appointed to the first pro-fessorship at Hopkins.

Many of the deficient schools, white schools as well as Black, were proprietary affairs, launched by individuals or small groups of physicians using funds from their own pockets or with help from churches or missionary societies. Some were purely commercial, conceived and run as money-making enterprises. Admissions standards were lax, often nonexistent, and facilities such as labo-ratories and libraries were substandard and frequently missing al-together. Haphazard courses of instruction and laissez-faire graduation standards flooded the country with practitioners who were not much more than doctors in name only. As medical his-torian Martin Kaufman points out, "The system inevitably re-sulted in hundreds of poorly educated doctors annually 'turned loose' upon an unsuspecting public."[7]

The low reputation and unpredictable competence of doctors inevitably led public authorities and medical organizations, the AMA in particular, to push for establishing professional standards that would raise the level of care and increase public trust in physicians, as well as elevate the social status of physicians, an especially sore issue for well-educated, competent practitioners. The AMA pushed for standards centered on medical schools, and an AMA committee began visiting schools and grading their curricula and the record of their graduates on state licensing exams. The AMA committee visited all of the country's medical schools and arrived at evaluations. But instead of publishing them, the AMA decided to ask a highly credible outside organization to conduct its own survey in order to have an objective confirmation of the AMA's conclusions. The association approached the Carnegie Foundation for the Advancement of Teaching, which launched a nationwide study in 1907 under the direction of Abraham Flexner.

Flexner was a teacher and educator who had studied classics at Johns Hopkins University and had done graduate work at Harvard and the University of Berlin. His book *The American College* had attracted the attention of the Carnegie Foundation's president, Henry Pritchett, who had also consulted with the director of the Rockefeller Institute for Medical Research—the pathologist Simon Flexner, Abraham's older brother. Simon Flexner had been a fellow, and then assistant professor of pathology at Johns Hopkins School of Medicine, where he was a protégé of William Welch. Abraham Flexner was an educational researcher and reformer. Though not a physician, he had close ties with Johns Hopkins and was fully aware, through his brother Simon, of its science-based approach to medical education. While studying in Germany he had also looked closely at the pedagogical practices of European universities and especially medical schools that had embraced the biomedical model championed by Rudolf Virchow and his students.

With that background, it was natural that Johns Hopkins was the first medical school Abraham Flexner visited as head of the Carnegie study. A close-up look at Hopkins—its facilities, its teaching hospital, and the superlative cast of founding professors William Welch had assembled—convinced Flexner of the direction all American schools ought to be taking. Flexner subsequently visited every medical school in the United States and Canada, but, he wrote later, "The rest of my study of medical education was little more than an amplification of what I had learned during my initial visit to Baltimore."[8]

Flexner needed little convincing. He had thought deeply about medical education and was well aware of the consensus among medical educators regarding the necessity of incorporating the biosciences into medical school curricula.[9] He was also knowledgeable about the general transformation of university studies that encompassed an approach to teaching and learning analogous to the new thinking about medical education. American education was entering a new, "progressive" era, rejecting the formalism of the lecture-and-memorization model and substituting a grounding in the basics that enabled experimentation, practical experience, and creative thinking. In medical schools, this meant science, laboratory work, and hands-on interaction with patients.[10]

Flexner visited 155 schools all told. It took him a year and a half of continuous travel and relentless work. His examinations were detailed and thorough. He looked at entrance requirements, number of students, number of instructors, budgets, laboratory facilities, and clinical facilities. All the schools he visited apparently opened their records for his examination, likely because, one historian conjectured, the name Carnegie created in the heads of desperate administrators "dancing visions of endowment plums."[11]

Abraham Flexner was an acute observer and a stern, objective critic who pulled no punches. "For twenty-five years past," Carnegie president Pritchett wrote in the report's introduction, "there has been an enormous over-production of uneducated and ill-trained medical practitioners. This has been in absolute disregard of public welfare. . . . Overproduction of ill-trained men is due in the main to the existence of a very large number of commercial schools, sustained in many cases by advertising methods through which a mass of unprepared youth is drawn out of industrial occupations into the study of medicine."[12]

In 1910 the Carnegie Foundation published Flexner's report (also known as *Carnegie Foundation Bulletin Number Four*). The period leading up to the report had already seen the closing of many precarious, underfunded, commercial schools that could not comply with increasingly strict state licensing requirements and had little ability to respond to the advances in the scientific understanding of disease. "These schools," writes sociologist Paul Starr, "were at the end of their tether; at that point it was relatively easy to strangle them."[13] Flexner's unsparing report did exactly that. It damned the schools whose inadequacies he saw as incompatible with the requirements for turning out competent doctors and in the process spelled an end to the free-wheeling, unregulated era of medical instruction and practice that went back to the beginning of the colonial experience.

Starting in 1907 Flexner visited 155 American and Canadian medical schools. By 1915 only ninety-five schools were still open. By 1930 that number had dropped to sixty-six. Among the schools that closed in the wake of the Flexner Report were five of the seven Black medical schools that had survived into the twentieth century (two of the three extant women's medical schools also closed). As these schools shut their doors, the sparse medical care of the South's largely rural Black population became even sparser.

The Flexner Report is widely seen as the most significant document in the history of American health care. But its effects, as beneficial as they have been in the professionalization of American medical schools and physicians and in the furtherance of the scientific spirit in medicine, were also negative. William Osler, the great Johns Hopkins clinician and later Oxford University clinician, came to believe that an overemphasis on the scientific understanding of disease channeled doctors' attention toward the disease per se rather than toward the patient. He feared, he said, that the model Welch was following would produce "a set of clinical prigs, the boundary of whose horizon would be the laboratory, and whose only human interest would be research."[14] Osler, Thomas Duffy writes, "placed the welfare of patients and the education of students to that effect as more important priorities."[15] One contemporary document, a letter to *Collier's* magazine by a doctor at a small medical school in Tennessee, expressed in intimate and personal (and distraught) terms the potential devastating results of the Flexner Report. While the writer may or may not have been Black, his words express the plight of the Black medical schools, the doctors who came out of them, and the patients they cared for: "True, our entrance requirements are not the same as those of the University of Pennsylvania or Harvard; nor do we pretend to turn out the same finished product. Yet we prepare worthy, ambitious men who have striven hard with small opportunities and risen above their surroundings to become family doctors to the farmers of the south. . . . Would you say that such people should be denied physicians?"[16]

Flexner had no time for this way of thinking. Of the seven Black medical schools—Howard, Meharry, Flint, Leonard, Knoxville, Louisville National, and West Tennessee—only two, he declared, were worth salvaging: Howard and Meharry. In his chapter "The Medical Education of the Negro," he wrote:

> Of the seven medical schools for negroes in the United States, five are at this moment in no position to make any contribution of value. . . . The upbuilding of Howard and Meharry will profit the nation much more than the inadequate maintenance of a larger number of schools. They are, of course, unequal to the need and the opportunity, but nothing will be gained by way of satisfying the need or of rising to the opportunity through the survival of feeble, ill-equipped institutions, quite regardless of the spirit that animates the promoters.

A parallel consequence of Flexner's report was the disappearance of all but one of the country's seven women's medical colleges that existed at the turn of the century.

Flexner's evaluations were brutally frank. According to medical historian Rosemary Stevens, "Twenty colleges were said to have closed in order that their conditions would not be described in the Flexner report."[17] It's understandable that may have happened; Flexner's reports could be brutal. Here's how Flexner described Flint Medical College in his general consideration that followed an enumeration of its resources: "Flint Medical College is a hopeless affair on which money and energy alike are wasted." About Knoxville Medical College he reported: "The catalogue of this school is a tissue of misrepresentations from cover to cover."

Flint and Knoxville, along with Louisville National, closed within a year or two of the publication of the Flexner Report. Leonard, the largest of the affected Black schools, lasted until 1918; West Tennessee, until 1923. Some students from these schools were able to continue their education at Meharry and Howard. For many, a career in medicine was a forlorn and eventually abandoned hope.

CHAPTER 4

AMHPS: The Founding

In the early fall of 1974, a meeting took place in a private room at New York City's Hilton Hotel. Nine men were present; two were white, seven Black. The white men were Pierre Galletti, vice president for medicine at Brown University, and Arthur Richardson, dean of the Emory University School of Medicine. The other seven were all connected with Morehouse College: Hugh Gloster, the president; Joseph Gayles, a professor; three board members; Bill Bennet, a consultant to Gloster from the National Institutes of Health; and Louis Wade Sullivan, a Morehouse alumnus who was a professor of medicine at Boston University. Gloster had called the group together and was presiding.

Morehouse, a historically Black college in Atlanta, had for more than a year been exploring the possibility of launching a medical school. Many who knew about the idea thought it little more than a fantasy. Morehouse College was highly regarded, but it was a small, liberal arts school with limited resources. Medical schools were notoriously expensive, troublesome institutions. Medical school professors drew higher salaries than those in other fields;

their research required specialized laboratories; they could be territorial, egotistical, and harder to manage than faculty at a traditional, well-ordered liberal arts college. But President Gloster was an energetic and optimistic man. He had been actively pursuing the medical school idea for a number of years, and in the last twelve months he had kicked planning into high gear. He had conducted a feasibility study. He had mobilized consultants and alumni and had driven the project forward, even though much of his constituency thought the idea quixotic, even dangerous to the health of the college.

But now the core groups that Gloster had put together were convinced that it could be done. Morehouse had a first-rate premed program, a large and loyal alumni organization, and strong leadership. It also had a certain mystique. President Gloster's predecessor, Benjamin Mays, had led Morehouse for almost thirty years. Mays was one of the founders of the civil rights movement. At Morehouse he had mentored Martin Luther King Jr., who called Mays his "intellectual father." Other major Black figures, including Maynard Jackson, Julian Bond, and others, had been his students. Mays was inspiring and charismatic. In his weekly chapel lectures, he told the undergraduates they could do anything they put their minds to. "The tragedy of life," he said, "isn't in failing to reach your goals, it's not having goals to reach." The attitude he had stamped on Morehouse's students had carried over to the college administrators and faculty. Morehouse had an ambitious, vigorous institutional culture—perhaps an outsized vision of its own capabilities. President Gloster was no less imbued with that mindset than his predecessor had been.

Many trustees, alumni, and faculty might have been skeptical of Gloster's plan, but at some level, the challenge engaged their pride in their school's can-do mentality. Given the right encouragement, even the skeptics could be brought on board, Gloster

thought. Beyond that, Gloster was sure the time was right for a
new Black medical school. Throughout the country, African American rates of disease and death were sky high compared to white
rates, worse in Georgia than most other places. African Americans
suffered far higher incidence of stroke, hypertension, cancer, and
other serious conditions and illnesses than did whites. The death
rate for Black infants was twice that for white infants. African
Americans lived, on average, five years less than whites did. There
was one white doctor for every 795 white Georgians. There was
one Black doctor for every 13,810 Black Georgians. Many Black
Georgians had virtually no access to health care. The need for
more Black physicians was dire.

The statistics were known. In 1967 the state had issued a *Physician Manpower* report that documented the extreme shortage of
all physicians in Georgia and the inability of Georgia's two medical schools to address the need. In the entire state, only ninety-five
Black doctors were practicing, and many were older and projected
to age out or die in the coming years. With a need so overwhelming, and now so public, the creation of a Black medical school that
would produce mostly primary care physicians couldn't have been
more pressing, or more obvious. In addition, the civil rights movement had put the case for Black equality front and center in the
country's consciousness, magnified in 1968 by the death of Martin Luther King. Gloster's project was taking shape at a critical moment in what seemed to be a propitious environment.

One of the groups Gloster had mustered to help plan and determine feasibility was an advisory committee of Morehouse
alumni who were in academic medicine. David Satcher, a research
scientist and family medicine specialist at Drew Postgraduate
School of Medicine and future surgeon general, was on the committee, as was Henry Foster a distinguished professor at Meharry
Medical College. Another was Louis Wade Sullivan, professor of

medicine at Boston University School of Medicine and future secretary of the Department of Health and Human Services under President George H. W. Bush.

Like others on the committee, Sullivan had initially been both intrigued and dubious. But, also like his colleagues, he had slowly come around to the idea that Morehouse might actually be able to do it. As he saw the possibilities, his enthusiasm grew, and after a year of meetings, he was all in. When he was asked to draw up a list of physicians he thought had the ability to handle the immense task of establishing and building a new medical school, he contemplated the limited number of African Americans in academic medicine and put together a list of ten individuals Gloster should consider. Later, he was surprised to get a phone call from Joseph Gayles, the Morehouse professor who was Gloster's point man. Gayles thanked Sullivan for the list but told him it was incomplete.

It took a moment before Sullivan realized that Gayles was saying he hadn't included his own name on his list of candidates. "Wait a minute," Sullivan said. "If you're talking about me, I'm not interested. I am *not* a candidate."

"Well," said Gayles. "We were hoping you'd at least be on the list, but I understand. If you're not interested, you're not interested. But . . . might I ask if you could come down to New York for a meeting. Not as a candidate, just as a consultant. We'd like your personal assessment of whether we should go forward."

So, in 1974, Sullivan was sitting with the others in the Hilton. For several hours they discussed the obstacles a new school would encounter and ideas for dealing with them. The committee asked what Sullivan thought about the qualities a founding dean should have. Sullivan was a well-known clinician, researcher, and teacher, the chief of Boston University's hematology service at Boston City Hospital. He knew his own dean well and he knew others at the Boston area's medical schools. He was well aware of what a dean's job entailed, its demands and some of its potential pitfalls. Years earlier, as a young professor he had been on the faculty of a promising new medical school at a prominent university, and had watched the school crash and burn. During Sullivan's time as a medical student, Boston University's own medical school had experienced such conflicts with the rest of the university that the dean had to cast around for another home and had found that such established and wealthy institutions as Princeton and MIT had no intention of taking on something as problematic as a medical school. Sullivan had a good understanding of the skills a dean would need just to survive, let alone flourish. He laid those out for the committee as clearly as he could, knowing they had a tough job in front of them. He knew that selecting the right person was going to take a lot of careful thought.

As the meeting drew to a close, President Gloster stood up. "First," he said to Sullivan, "I want to thank you for coming down and helping us clarify our thoughts. I know, of course, you're here as a consultant, not as a candidate. Now," he paused a moment, "I can't speak for the committee, but I do want to tell you that in my own mind, you are just the person we're looking for. I hope you'll give it serious consideration."

On the drive back from New York to Boston that evening, Sullivan asked his wife, Ginger, a native New Englander, "Do you think you might possibly consider moving to Atlanta?" "I knew it," she said. "I just knew it!" Six months later, on April 2, 1975, Sullivan was in Atlanta being introduced to the media as the founding dean of the new Morehouse School of Medicine.

Sullivan hadn't made his decision easily. Friends had warned him about the dangers and potential for catastrophic failure. "It's a crazy idea," one had said. "Don't do it." But despite the warnings, he had decided to accept. The reason he had went back to his own early life in Blakely, a small town in the southwest corner of Georgia.

Neither Blakely nor any of the surrounding towns had had a Black doctor. If African Americans in Blakely were sick enough to need medical attention, their options were limited. They could do without and let nature take its course; they could go to one of the local root doctors—folk healers who dealt in roots and herbs, potions and magic spells; or they could go to the white doctor. But seeing the white doctor meant going around back and sitting in a separate waiting room. It meant acquiescing to the so-called universal presumption of Black inferiority. People considered it demeaning, an affront, one among the constant stream of affronts that conditioned their lives in Jim Crow Blakely.

The Black doctor nearest to Blakely was Joseph Griffin, who ran a clinic and private hospital in Bainbridge, forty miles away. Dr. Griffin was famous throughout southern Georgia. There was no one more respected in the Black community. Sullivan's father knew Dr. Griffin well. As a funeral director in Blakely, the elder Sullivan had one of the few Black-owned cars in town—his hearse. If someone needed to see Dr. Griffin, Mr. Sullivan drove them there, often taking his son along for the ride. Dr. Griffin—in his green scrubs, taking care of the sick, often healing them—had been Lou Sullivan's role model from the age of five. He had never wanted to be anything but a doctor like Dr. Griffin. When one of his professors at BU Medical School had asked what his future plans were, he told her he was going to go back to Georgia to practice family medicine.

It hadn't worked out that way. Sullivan had been seduced by the excitement of medical science and had gotten sidetracked by the world of hematology, a subspecialty of internal medicine. As a result, his earlier aspiration had long ago slipped away. But the Morehouse School of Medicine, if it worked, would eventually be graduating a stream of Black primary care physicians, and many would locate in the ghettos and the underserved—or unserved—rural reaches of the state. In a sense this was Sullivan's second chance at fulfilling his youthful ambition, but in an exponentially more-powerful way. That thought had tipped the scales.

~

Gloster had started his campaign for a new Black medical school in the early 1970s, but the original idea went back more than fifty years to Morehouse's first Black president, John Hope, who served from 1906 to 1929. It was a visionary aspiration, especially for that time. The 1910 Flexner Report on medical education had established the science-based curriculum of the Johns Hopkins University School of Medicine as the national standard and had led to the closing of many schools in the United States and Canada because they had inadequate laboratory, faculty, and other resources, and had no possibility of upgrading themselves. Of the seven Black medical schools functioning in 1910, five had closed their doors by 1915; another held out until 1923. Only two Black schools met the Flexner Report standards and survived: Howard and Meharry, which meant that Hope had conceptualized his endeavor against a forbidding background of school closures and vastly increased financial requirements.

Hope might have been a visionary, but he was also a determined, persistent pragmatist. An educator and political activist, he was a close associate of W. E. B. Du Bois in founding the Niagara Movement, predecessor of the National Association for the Advancement of Colored People (NAACP), and an important figure in the Urban League and other civil rights organizations. He had become president of Morehouse College in 1906, when it still had its earlier name, Atlanta Baptist College, and he guided Morehouse as its president for twenty-three years.

Hope was the fourth president of Morehouse, and the first African American to hold the office. Together with his lifelong friend Du Bois, Hope emphasized the importance of training Black professionals for roles as leaders in the African American community and for achievement in both public and private spheres, a concept that Du Bois popularized as "The Talented Tenth." Black education, both Du Bois and Hope believed, should emphasize the traditional arts and sciences at the college level and beyond.

Hope had been a classics professor before his appointment as Morehouse president; he was especially focused on making graduate school education available to Black students. To further that objective, he proposed that Atlanta's five Black colleges—Atlanta University, Morehouse College, Spelman College, Clark College, and Morris Brown College—should merge into one institution. It was an idea that had occurred to him years earlier, and by the 1920s he had fleshed out the concept. Given the aggregate resources, Hope believed the schools could form one strong university rather than five struggling colleges, a university incorporating undergraduate and graduate programs and professional schools, including a school of medicine. In his vision, Atlanta University would become the graduate component of the unified institution, fed by undergraduates from the other college components. The merger proposal met with stiff opposition partly because the schools had different religious affiliations and partly because many alumni were appalled by the prospect of losing their alma mater's identity.

Hope wasn't easily discouraged though. In 1925 the Claremont College consortium had been founded in California made up of several small colleges organized along the lines of Oxford University and its various component colleges. In 1929 Hope proposed a similar consortium structure for Atlanta's Black institutions.

This time he had more luck. That same year the five schools formed a consortium (Atlanta University Center Consortium), and Hope's proposal that Atlanta University become a graduate rather than an undergraduate institution was accepted. Two years later, in 1931, Hope gave up the presidency of Morehouse to become president of Atlanta University to focus his attention on graduate education. Even before moving over to Atlanta University, he recruited Dr. Marque Jackson, an African American physician in Chicago, to work toward establishing a medical school.

Jackson hadn't gone far, though, before the stock market crashed, bringing the Great Depression in its wake. Given the crippling economic and social consequences, Hope told Jackson they would have to put the project off for a while. But in 1936 Hope died, and his idea was shelved. Now, fifty years after Hope's initial effort, Morehouse College's seventh president, Hugh Gloster, brought the concept back to life.

President Gloster had various reasons for thinking the times might favor a new Black medical school. In the years between John Hope's presidency and his own, the county's thinking about race had evolved. In 1948 Harry Truman had ended segregation in the armed forces, at the same time banning discrimination in the federal work force. In front of the Lincoln Memorial, Truman had told NAACP delegates, "It is my deep conviction that we have reached a turning point in the long history of our country's efforts to guarantee freedom and equality to all our citizens."[1]

In the years following Truman's presidency, one dramatic event after another focused the nation's attention on the issue of racial equality: the Montgomery bus boycott, *Brown v. Board of Education*, sit-ins, freedom rides, Selma, Alabama. The pressure mounted. Black heroes emerged on the national scene: Rosa Parks, Thurgood Marshall, Martin Luther King Jr. Then in 1964 the landmark

Civil Rights Act became law, ending segregation in public places and in employment, followed in 1965 by the Voting Rights Act, which erased the Jim Crow local laws that prevented Blacks from voting.

The civil rights movement had put the case for Black equality front and center in the nation's consciousness. When Gloster was named Morehouse president in 1967, the issue of Black equality was a burning concern. Then came the tremendous shock of King's assassination, which riveted the country's attention like little else before it. Gloster's desire to start a primarily Black medical school thus began taking shape at a critical historic moment. Almost a hundred years after the end of Reconstruction, the country was beginning to come to terms with its legacy of slavery, segregation, and prejudice.

One of those legacies was the abysmal state of Black health and health care. In the final decades of the nineteenth century, the idea had taken root that Black mortality and morbidity rates were so bad that African American citizens were headed for extinction. While no one thought that any longer in the 1970s, Black babies and mothers were still dying at much faster rates than white mothers and babies, African American adults had shorter life spans, and the most dangerous diseases and conditions manifested among Blacks at significantly higher rates than among whites.

For anyone aware of these disparities, at the top of the list of reasons why this was so was the drastic shortage of African American physicians nationwide. "Of all the forms of inequality," Martin Luther King had said, "injustice in health is the most shocking and inhuman."[2] Almost nowhere was that truer than in the state of Georgia. Even in the face of hardened segregationist opposition, health conditions for Blacks demanded at least some attention. For Hugh Gloster, that encouraged him to think the time was right for a new medical school that would add to the flow of African American primary care physicians.

Gloster also saw a window of opportunity in the amount of federal money available for medical school construction and salaries—although that window was closing quickly. Projections about the substantial number of doctors needed in the United States had led in 1963 to the Health Professions Educational Assistance Act and its follow-ups. That and other federal and state funding sources had stimulated the development of new medical schools to help meet the projected physician shortages. From late 1965 until the early 1970s, twenty-five new medical schools had opened their doors. But Congress was beginning to believe that the manpower requirements had now not only been met, but that the spike in building and expansion might even produce a surplus. As a result, the generous federal funding seemed headed for retrenchment. Gloster wanted to get the medical school project up and running while the funds were still available.

In 1973 Gloster pushed his initiative into high gear. He received a Bureau of Manpower grant from the Public Health Service to do a feasibility study, and he organized committees to study needs, funding, organization, and other aspects of establishing a school of medicine. Gloster also had important outside help. Emory University and Emory School of Medicine were located in Atlanta, and the medical school's dean, Arthur Richardson, worked with Gloster to develop his plans. In the wake of the civil rights movement, white medical schools were attempting to recruit Black students. But the best Black undergraduates were going to schools like Johns Hopkins, Harvard and Stanford, which meant that Emory, without the same scholarship resources or level of prestige, was having a hard time attracting African American applicants. To compensate and help fulfill what he considered Emory's obligation, Dean Richardson did what he could to support Gloster's medical project. In the Atlanta health world, nothing was more important than Emory's cooperation.

Both Louis Brown, chairman of the state's Black National Medical Association chapter, and Rhodes Haverty, chairman of Georgia's white AMA chapter, also committed their organizations to the project, which is especially interesting since historically the AMA had prohibited Black doctors from joining and had erected barriers to their professional lives. But now Georgia's white and Black doctors banded together to support the Morehouse medical school endeavor.

Louis Brown was an especially zealous advocate. He himself had played a leading role in introducing the idea of a medical school into Gloster's thinking. Back in 1967, the year Gloster was named president, the Georgia Department of Public Health had issued a *Physician Manpower* report that highlighted the state's extreme shortage of doctors, including Black doctors. Brown, an Atlanta family physician, was one of Georgia's shockingly small number of Black practitioners. He had been cochair of the committee that had written the *Physician Manpower* report, and when it came out he had brought the idea for a new medical school to the consortium's presidents, including the newly appointed Hugh Gloster. Brown had proposed that Atlanta University establish a school, but after a blue ribbon outside committee found such an endeavor beyond Atlanta's capability, the University had declined to move ahead. With that, Gloster had taken up the cause.

When Gloster asked Sullivan to head the new school, he had not known about Sullivan's early desire to return to Georgia after medical school as a family physician. But now the proposed Morehouse School of Medicine offered the possibility of fulfilling his early dream, many times over, by producing an ongoing supply of primary care doctors, a good percentage of whom would be establishing practices in Georgia's impoverished African American communities and neighborhoods.

~

The challenges and excitement of building a medical school from scratch absorbed Sullivan completely: hiring faculty and administrators, making building plans and renting space, finding public and private funding sources, developing a meaningful curriculum, and publicizing the new school. Morehouse School of Medicine was launched in 1975 (until 1977 it was, technically, the Medical Education Program at Morehouse College). The first hurdle was getting conditional accreditation, only then could they begin attracting students. Sullivan made steady progress on all fronts, but one problem troubled him deeply.

He'd been invited to an early meeting with the executive committee of the National Medical Association board and had expected a cordial welcome. Instead he had found himself in a chilly atmosphere, facing a group of serious men asking serious questions. The majority of the committee members were graduates of either Howard or Meharry, and for most of the twentieth century, the world of Black medical schools had consisted of only these two institutions. The committee members made clear to Sullivan their deep misgivings about a third school, which would cut into the available pool of federal funding. A third school might be a positive in terms of increasing the flow of African American physicians, but wouldn't Morehouse pose a threat to their own funding? This was a zero-sum game. What was Dr. Sullivan's answer to that?

Sullivan had ducked and weaved around that question. But the fact was he had no answer to it, and as he built his school, it stayed on his mind. Meharry and Howard were natural allies of Morehouse in the urgent need to produce Black doctors and in the overarching need to improve the abysmal state of Black health. It made no sense for them to regard each other as competitors. But what could bring the three schools together as allies rather than as rivals to pursue their mutual interests?

As Sullivan considered this question, several experiences led him toward an answer. One was the capitation funding he had succeeded in getting from the state of Georgia. Capitation funding meant that the state had agreed to provide financial support based on the number of enrolled students, the expectation being that many would be going into primary care in Georgia. Another new medical school—Mercer School of Medicine—had opened in Georgia shortly after Morehouse did. It was a mainline school, attracting mostly white students. Like Morehouse, Mercer School of Medicine was also avidly seeking capitation funds.

To push for this funding from the state legislature, Morehouse supporters and Mercer supporters joined forces. Both schools—Morehouse in Atlanta and Mercer in Macon, near the geographic center of the state—gathered support from their alumni and from local political figures and legislators. The two schools and their supporters were obvious partners; together they brought significantly more clout to the legislative battle than either would have been able to bring by itself.

That experience had Sullivan thinking about the potential influence that Howard, Meharry, and Morehouse together—in alliance—might have in funding and minority health issues in Congress. Howard in Washington, DC, Meharry in Tennessee, and Morehouse in Georgia each had vocal alumni. Meharry and Morehouse played political roles in their states, especially since the Voting Rights Act had enlarged Black political power. Washington, DC, had no real legislative representation, but Howard had connections and a degree of influence in the capital. How much more powerful the three voices together would be, Sullivan thought; they could better leverage their power if they acted as one.

Additionally, Sullivan's early experience with public funding made him think that *multiple* government sources might be available, if only one knew how to effectively tap them. He had been awarded state funding through a couple of different avenues. The medical school had also received an unsolicited grant from the commissioners of Fulton County, which included the city of Atlanta. Fulton County was responsible for health in its district. One of the newly elected commissioners was a Morehouse alumnus who had graduated several years after Sullivan and who saw Morehouse School of Medicine as furthering the county's health agenda. These experiences awakened Sullivan to the potential for significant public support using different points of leverage.

With some degree of thought, preparation, and coordination, Morehouse School of Medicine, Sullivan believed, was positioned to get significant public funding from various federal, state, and local governmental entities. And if Morehouse could do that on its own, what could they do if they had on their side congressional representatives from Tennessee and the clout within the Capitol that Howard could bring? And what if they could also tie in other Black health institutions which would bring with them their own supporters and legislators?

Sullivan's initial talks with Howard University did not go well. Howard had a special subsidy arrangement with Congress that went back to 1879 but had to be reapproved every year. The university had no interest in drawing unwanted attention to this badly needed money stream by engaging in lobbying efforts for other federal funding. So the answer from Howard, the senior Black medical institution, was no.

Sullivan's discussion with Meharry's president, Lloyd Elam, went differently. Elam was receptive. The idea sounded worth pursuing. Meharry was under financial stress, and an association that might strengthen the school's efforts to attract funding was welcome. Two years earlier at the NMA's executive committee meeting, Meharry's board chair had expressed his reservations about Morehouse. But President Elam brought a different perspective. He was an academic, like Sullivan. Both men were thinking only of the upside.

Meharry, it turned out, already had a working relationship of sorts with the Xavier University College of Pharmacy in New Orleans and Tuskegee School of Veterinary Medicine in Tuskegee, Alabama. The three schools were in discussion together about obtaining federal construction loans. As a result, Sullivan now found himself talking with Xavier's president, Norman Francis, and Tuskegee veterinary school dean Walter Bowie, along with Elam, proposing to all of them a formal alliance that would enhance their ability to influence congressional policies on minority health and legislation that would benefit all their institutions.

In the fall of 1977 Sullivan hosted the first meeting of what was to become the Association of Minority Health Professions Schools (AMHPS). The principals met in Atlanta at the Morehouse School of Medicine, where Sullivan's offices were still in the double-wide trailers he and Gloster had rented as temporary medical school space. At that meeting the concept of an association was fleshed out, together with discussion about the issues the group should focus on. Sullivan's initial thinking included a vision of the association as a kind of Brookings Institution, conducting research on issues and making policy recommendations. While all the participants were well aware of the dearth of research on Black health, they knew that at this juncture their priority was to identify the issues that most demanded attention, issues that they could forge into a platform of sorts as they decided how best to publicize their concerns and pursue congressional action.

Xavier University College of Pharmacy, meanwhile, had institutional connections with the country's two other historically Black pharmacy schools, Florida A&M and Texas Southern University, and they too joined the association. When the Charles Drew Postgraduate School of Medicine came aboard shortly afterward, all of the major American Black health schools, with the exception of Howard, were now affiliated with each other in a way no one had previously envisioned.

This seemed to Sullivan and the other presidents and deans a natural evolution, emerging out of the advantages they saw in speaking with a single voice in the halls of power. The acute shortage of African American health professionals was a lead factor in the appalling state of Black health nationwide. The schools were far too few, their finances fragile, the legacy of prejudice and discrimination still a barrier to the professional advancement of their graduates, even in the new post–civil rights, post–Martin Luther King world. But all of them saw the late 1970s as a time of opportunity. Together they marshaled significant strengths—the commitment of their administrators, the professional qualifications of their faculties, and perhaps most significantly, the political leverage they could bring to bear in this new era of Black rights.

A new development in the congressional arena was also working in their favor. Only a few years before, the small but militant group of Black representatives had banded together as the Congressional Black Caucus (CBC). With them, the nascent association had a core of committed, energetic legislators on their side, in particular Louis Stokes, the first Black representative from Ohio. Stokes was one of the founders of the CBC, and in the late 1970s he and his colleagues set up what they called "Brain Trusts," working groups that identified issues of importance to the Black community and recommended possible legislative action. There was a Housing Brain Trust, a Small Business Brain Trust, and a Health

Brain Trust, which Stokes headed. Stokes's commitment to African American health issues went back to his first term in Congress a decade earlier. Now, as the only Black member of the House Appropriations Committee, he wielded considerable power. Stokes and Sullivan had forged a close working relationship going back to 1975, shortly after the founding of Morehouse School of Medicine. Here, then, with Stokes, Ralph Metcalf, Bill Clay, and other members of the caucus, was a power base inside the legislature.

The white world too was opening up. AMHPS had natural allies in congressmen like Arlen Specter, Paul Rogers, Tom Harkins, and Warren Magnuson. Sullivan had also cultivated relations with Georgia's two senators, Sam Nunn and Herman Talmadge, both warmly receptive to the aims of the new Black organization. Talmadge's support was a phenomenon in itself, an indicator of which way the winds were blowing. Talmadge's father, Eugene Talmadge, had been a fire-eating, "segregation now, segregation tomorrow, segregation forever" governor. Herman Talmadge himself had been a diehard opponent of the Civil Rights Act, one of a group of Southern senators who fought tooth and nail against equal rights and the encroachment of integration in the old, white supremacist South. But in the 1970s, with African Americans voting in ever-larger numbers, Talmadge began to shift his positions on race, trying hard to put his past behind him. Support of efforts to improve Black health care was an avenue to that end; even among segregationists, few could condemn endeavors to improve health. Strom Thurmond himself, the leading prosegregation figure of his time, became a supporter of AMHPS's efforts.

With the political landscape changing, the stark health disparities between Blacks and the mainstream white population began to emerge as a national issue in a way it never had before. Earlier there had been an awareness of Black vulnerability to disease and death and speculation about why that should be, much of it racist in nature, little of it in terms of what might be done to ameliorate it. But now some congressmen and other public figures were viewing disparities through the lens of civil rights and the commitment, as President Truman had put it, "to guarantee equality to all our citizens." Some portion of white America, at least, was understanding disparities in health care and outcomes from a moral perspective.

Black doctors had always seen it that way, and now Sullivan, Elam, and their colleagues were preparing to take on this particular miscarriage of justice through legislative means. Disparities in health care meant, in plain language, more Black sickness and more Black death. In broad terms, it meant Black Americans lives were simply worth less than white lives. What then should be done to strengthen the institutions whose graduates were the backbone of minority health care? Sullivan, Elam, and their colleagues intended to answer that question. The conscience of the society in terms of racial equality had risen to a level not seen before. With AMHPS, the mobilization of Black institutional resources was also something new on the American health care scene.

~

By the beginning of the 1980s, AMHPS's leaders had gone a long way toward defining the association's role and its priorities. As AMHPS readied itself to engage with Congress on health care legislation, the member institutions incorporated, turning their informal affiliation into a legal entity.

> The name of the corporation shall be the Association of Minority
> Health Professions Schools.
>
> The purpose of this corporation shall be to assist its member
> institutions individually and collectively in their efforts to expand
> and improve educational opportunities in the health professions for
> minority and disadvantaged persons, to increase the number of

minority health personnel, to improve access to health care for minority and disadvantaged persons, and to undertake the measures necessary to improve the health status of minority and disadvantaged persons.

By now it was also clear to the principals that they needed to document the issues they had been discussing: the disparities, the shortages of Black health care professionals, the needs of the training institutions, the preparation of minority students for careers in health care, the significance of Black health care for the larger society, the ongoing barriers against inclusion. Rather than simply going in and talking to legislators, they needed a document that would define the issues concisely and provide evidence that was not only anecdotal but drawn from research, a document that legislators and staffers could use in making their own case for these issues to others. They had to be able to present the hard data that would support their efforts to educate and would provide a rationale for their proposals.

From acquaintances in Washington, Sullivan heard that with the Carter administration coming to an end, Ruth Hanft, deputy assistant HHS secretary for health policy and research, was leaving her job and might be available to work for AMHPS. Hanft was known for her research skills and lucid, disciplined writing. In short order, she was hired and went to work compiling the statistics and reportage that was to serve as a white paper for the association.

AMHPS also took the crucial step of finding a Washington lobbyist and advocate. Back when Sullivan had started looking at the possibilities of government funding for Morehouse School of Medicine, a friend had told him, "You need someone who understands who's who in the legislature, what their relationships are, what their motives are, and how you can maneuver them. You need a lobbyist." Sullivan had hired a lobbyist to act for him in Georgia and also a Washington, DC, attorney who specialized in educational institutions. Now Sullivan's Washington attorney, Ray Cotton, recommended the Health and Medicine Counsel, a lobbying firm whose founder, Harley Dirks, had been chief of staff for Senator Warren Magnuson, one of Congress's leading proponents of health care.

The board was now meeting quarterly, fine-tuning its thinking about the issues and its priorities. The principals attended, the presidents and deans, along with consultants they called in, and also with Ruth Hanft, listening and taking notes as the discussions progressed. They wanted Hanft there, not just to document the proceedings but to get a personal feel for the institutions she would be writing about—their history, the problems they faced, their fragility, and their significance. They needed to present the hard facts and figures, but they also wanted to project their sense of urgency.

Hanft was in her fifties, a veteran health care policy specialist, and a chain smoker in an era when smoking was still acceptable in public places, except that reports were starting to appear about the dangers of smoking and even of inhaling secondhand smoke. Chain smoking for Hanft meant that as one cigarette burned down, she used the stub to light the next. As a result, health care discussions often went on in a haze of tobacco smoke that gave all the doctors sitting at the table a strong dose of secondhand-smoke exposure. At one point David Satcher, who by then was president of Meharry Medical College, finally moved that "meetings of the board shall henceforth be smoke free." (Both Satcher, the future surgeon general, and Sullivan, the future Health and Human Services secretary, were to make anti-smoking campaigns a priority.) Satcher's motion carried unanimously, which cleared the air but also prolonged the meetings as Hanft had to step outside regularly to light up and take a few long drags.

Her smoking habit, though, did nothing to affect her research and writing. In the spring of 1983 Hanft's 121-page paper was ready. It was titled *Blacks and the Health Professions in the '80s: A National Crisis and a Time for Action*. Its stated purpose was: "To describe the health status of the black population and the role of the black health professional; to describe the role of the minority schools in educating black health professionals; to raise policy issues, and to offer policy options."

Here were succinct summaries of the state of Black health, of Black health care professionals, of minority schools and their financing, of students and faculty—placed in their historical context, describing the present reality, projecting the future, supported by tables, spelling out the issues, and describing the options. It was exactly what the AMHPS principals, staff, and lobbyists needed to mount their case for the crucial expansion of congressional support for their institutions.

Although no one from AMHPS could have predicted it, the Hanft report turned out to be a historic, vastly consequential document. AMHPS leaders thought of it as a compendium of facts that substantiated their arguments, a helpful supporting document as they looked for public exposure and began their lobbying efforts. But it turned out to be a great deal more. The Hanft report was the first time anyone had ever brought together the facts about the extreme nationwide shortage of Black health professionals as it related to the dire health of the Black population. The report opened a new avenue of thinking about disparities in health care, research on Black health, and potential legislative cures for the injustices and inequities that had plagued Black health care since Black health had first become any kind of issue in the wake of emancipation. It's not too much to say that the Hanft report precipitated many of the essential changes in the treatment of minorities and women that have materialized in the thirty-nine years since its release.

Once the new report was ready, the next step was to introduce it and get some exposure where it counted. For that they enlisted the help of Judy Miller Jones who directed the Health Policy Forum at George Washington University. Jones set up a press conference at the National Press Club, and then symposia and other events for congressmen, staffers, and policy people at various Washington venues, creating an aura of interest in Black health care issues and in the new association of Black schools.

As AMHPS was getting itself onto the radar screen of policy experts and congressional staff, the association's leaders were thinking of the most likely pathways into the legislative process. One obvious first step would be to meet with Margaret Heckler, the recently appointed secretary of Health and Human Services. HHS was responsible for the National Institutes of Health, the country's major funder of medical research. The number of health care professionals—doctors, nurses, dentists, and others—was an HHS concern. HHS controlled the CDC, social security, and welfare. The HHS secretary could be a crucial figure in furthering AMHPS's objectives.

Or possibly not. Ronald Reagan had slashed educational funding essential to Black and other poor medical students. Reagan policies had damaged or eliminated other programs important to the African American community. Heckler was a Reagan appointee. Once Sullivan succeeded in arranging a meeting, his anxieties mounted. How would Heckler respond? Would she be indifferent, maybe even dismissive? Would she listen politely, then disregard what they would be presenting to her? Would she have any interest at all?

Heckler was from Massachusetts. When she was in Congress she had been on the moderate side, as far as Republicans went, but President Reagan had appointed her only a month earlier. There was a good chance that demonstrating loyalty would be high on her list of priorities. As Sullivan, David Satcher from Meharry Medical College, Walter Bowie from Tuskegee, and Alfred Haynes from Drew prepared to see Heckler, none of them had any confidence about how this meeting was likely to go.

CHAPTER 5

The Heckler Report

HHS Secretary Margaret Heckler knew something about the dismally inadequate number of Black students in medical schools. She had served in Congress from a Boston-area district from 1967 until a few months before the AMHPS leaders met with her in 1983. As a congresswoman, many of Heckler's constituents were affiliated with Boston's medical schools, and during her tenure the subject of Black medical school enrollment had ignited a vigorous and sometimes heated conversation in Boston's medical establishment.

The assassination of Martin Luther King Jr. had precipitated this conversation. King's murder in 1968 had been a cathartic moment, propelling racial prejudice to the forefront of public discussions. Boston's medical schools, along with many others in the country, had turned their attention to their long-observed practice of admitting only token numbers of Black students. At Harvard that number was three a year. At Boston University there were seven students of color in the entire school. These sorts of quotas had always been accepted as normal. But now there was a spotlight shining on the injustice they represented. One result was that professors at Boston University School of Medicine organized a New England–wide admissions forum for potential African American applicants from the South. Almost all New England medical schools signed on and welcomed the visiting students, who all received admission offers. This process was in high gear not long into Heckler's tenure, so she was aware of the issue.

The MLK-generated argument about increasing the numbers of Black medical students was all about injustice, inequality, and the benefits of diversity. The crying need for more Black doctors in impoverished areas of the South was not part of the discussion going on around Heckler's ears in Boston. So while Heckler knew something about Black medical students, she was not attuned to the presentation she was about to hear from Louis Sullivan, David Satcher, Walter Bowie, and Alfred Haynes.

The four leaders themselves were more than a little nervous as they walked into the massive Health and Human Services building designed by Marcel Breuer. None of them had spent much time in Washington, DC; they weren't on familiar ground. Although one or two had had some previous contacts with federal officials, this was the first time they were making a joint effort in the name of their association. In a sense, this was AMHPS's maiden voyage. A positive response from the secretary could have significant benefits, but that, they knew, was far from assured. They were fully prepared to listen to platitudes, then get a polite brush off.

In Heckler's offices they were shown into a conference room, then Heckler came in and greeted them cordially, putting them at ease. Sullivan introduced himself and the three others and thanked her for inviting them. He talked briefly about the institutions they represented, then launched into the essence of the report they were carrying with them. They were there, he said,

because the health and longevity of American Blacks was far be-
low the health and longevity of white Americans. Black Americans had a much heavier burden of illness. Black infant mortality
was twice that of white babies. Black adults died on average five
years earlier than white Americans. One of the leading reasons
for this situation was the severe shortage of Black physicians,
dentists, and other health professionals. "The schools we represent," he said, "are working as hard as we can to address this
truly dire situation. But in order to make any real dent in the problem, we need help and support from the federal government."

Satcher, Bowie, and Haynes added their own comments, and
then Sullivan handed Heckler the Hanft report, its subtitle *A National Crisis and a Time for Action.* "We've put together this report,"
he said. "It provides the data we've accumulated that shows spe-
cifics of these problems we've been talking about. We'd like to
leave it with you and to assure you that we are prepared to work
with you to address these concerns. We're eager to have your
thoughts and suggestions and, of course, the support of your
office."

Heckler took the 121-page report and leafed through it. "Thank
you," she said. "This looks quite impressive. I'll be reviewing it
carefully with my staff. You'll be hearing back from us."

The entire meeting took thirty-five minutes. As they walked out
of the building, the AMHPS leaders didn't know what to make of
what had just transpired. Heckler had been friendly, but that could
have been mostly for show. She had said she would look carefully
at the report, which sounded like it might have been bureaucra-
tese for, "Thanks; I'll look at this when and if I ever have the time."
None of them thought it a sure thing that she actually would get
back to them.

A month went by, then two months, then three, with no word
from Heckler's office. Heckler obviously had a full agenda, and

giant bureaucracies are by nature slow to shift attention to new subjects. It also wasn't clear how much power Heckler actually had, and if she was even capable of doing anything significant to help them, assuming that she wanted to. Except for the military, Ronald Reagan was tightening the federal budget every way he could. He had cut back on social welfare programs, cuts that had disproportionately impacted Black Americans. He had drastically reduced the National Health Service Corps scholarship program that all the Black institutions relied on heavily. He had very publicly supported Bob Jones University in its prohibition of cross-racial dating. Reagan's actions regarding race weren't encouraging. It was clear to the four AMHPS leaders that Reagan was looking to rein in the HHS budget not expand it and certainly not in regard to Black health institutions.

As the months passed with only silence from Heckler's office, the four men's hopes faded. They hadn't had high expectations of success to begin with, but that wasn't a great comfort as time went by, and it seemed more and more as if the urgent message they had tried to convey about the critical situation in Black health care had fallen on stony ground.

On the other hand, they weren't simply holding their breath waiting for a response. They were all running institutions that demanded more than full-time attention. Sullivan's new medical school was about to graduate its first class of MDs. He was pushing to increase foundation support and to recruit faculty, and was still working out the start-up administrative kinks. It had been less than a year since Morehouse School of Medicine had become independent of Morehouse College, and some of their facilities were still in rented space at the college, which wasn't ideal. Meanwhile, David Satcher had been brought in as president of Meharry in 1982 to try to rescue the school from oblivion. Meharry was dealing with a massive debt burden that the school could not repay and was on the verge of losing its accreditation because of inadequate faculty resources and the lack of hospital space. The *New York Times* had already announced Meharry's imminent demise. Satcher was wrestling with a life-and-death crisis. By 1983 it looked as if he might have turned the tide, but that wasn't yet assured. He harbored hopes that the secretary might do them some good, but Margaret Heckler was not at the very top of his concerns. The other presidents, Bowie at Tuskegee School of Veterinary Medicine and Hayes at Drew College of Medicine were dealing with their own difficult problems.

~

Six months after the meeting, there was still no response and no indication that one might be on the way. Had Heckler simply dismissed their concerns as not worth following up on? Or could there possibly be some kind of unresolved fight going on within the administration about how to deal with Black health issues and this new Black association? The AMHPS leaders didn't know. Nor did they know that Heckler's own staff opposed taking action on their report, and that she was fighting with them about it.[1] What they did know was that they had given Heckler their best shot, and it apparently had come to nothing.

Then, in April 1984, more than a year after their meeting, Sullivan received a letter from Secretary Heckler's office. The secretary, the letter said, had appointed a task force to investigate the health problems of minority Americans and the disparities in illness and death rates between whites and minorities. A list of committee members was attached to the letter. Heckler had appointed Tom Malone, deputy director of NIH, to chair the committee.

Seeing Malone's name gave Sullivan a momentary jolt of optimism, as it did Satcher and the others when he called to tell them that Heckler had finally responded. Tom Malone was a PhD biologist from Harvard University. He had been at NIH since the 1960s. Sullivan had interacted with him various times about research grants that Morehouse's faculty members were pursuing, as well as about other medical school matters. Sullivan's AMHPS colleagues also knew Malone, by reputation if not personally. Malone was highly respected. At NIH he was the chief administrator under director James Wyngaarden. Malone was the one who made the NIH trains run on time. He was also the highest ranking African American there.

Sullivan scanned the list of committee members to see whether there were any other African Americans. He saw Betty Lou Dotson's name. He had heard of her, although they had never met. Dotson was chief of the NIH Office for Civil Rights. Clay Simpson was also there. Sullivan hadn't met him either, although he knew Simpson was involved with medical education programs. But it turned out David Satcher knew him well. Simpson had been an active supporter of Meharry for years. He would be a strong ally. Donald Hopkins was also on the list. A tropical disease expert from the Bahamas, Hopkins was the deputy director of the CDC. Like Malone, Hopkins occupied a prominent position, although he had less of a public presence.

Toward the end of the list was Clarice Reid's name. Sullivan knew Reid. She was a sickle cell specialist in the NIH's Heart Lung and Blood Institute. When Sullivan was a professor at Boston University, he had helped establish a national sickle cell program, and Reid was a prominent part of the program. Now she was on her way to being named head of the NIH blood disease section. Satcher also knew her from the sickle cell program.

It seemed to the four leaders that Heckler had indeed read their report. Appointing Tom Malone was a signal that the secretary was taking their issues seriously. That gave them some cautious optimism. They didn't know how Malone was planning to run the task force or conduct the research. They couldn't even guess at what his conclusions might be or what sort of recommendations, if any, might come out of the investigation. They didn't want to get their hopes up. How many government reports had there been that never resulted in anything concrete? But the signs were pointing in the right direction. Malone was chairing. Dotson, Simpson, Hopkins, and Reid were on the committee. That could hardly have been an accident. Each of the presidents began to think that maybe this could actually end up with something significant.

It had taken a year for Heckler to move ahead and appoint her task force. It took another year for the task force to produce their report. When it was ready, Heckler asked the AMHPS leaders to come in. Tom Malone's letter to Heckler introducing the completed report put his committee's effort in its historical context: "Dear Madame Secretary . . . this report is a landmark effort in analyzing and synthesizing the present state of knowledge of the major factors that contribute to the health status of Blacks, Hispanics, Asian / Pacific Islanders and Native Americans. It represents the first time the Department of Health and Human Services has consolidated minority health issues into one report."

"This report," he went on, "should serve not only as a standard resource for department wide strategy, but as a generating force for an accelerated national assault on the persistent health disparities which led you to establish the Task Force a little more than a year ago." "One of the priority areas," Malone wrote, was "the development of health professionals that cut across all health problem areas." This, he said, "merited intensive action."

In Malone's letter the AMHPS leaders heard a ringing affirmation of the case they had made in the report they had left with the secretary two and a half years earlier. Malone's letter spoke of the persistent disparities and the need to develop more Black health

professionals, precisely the chief concern and mission of their institutions. He was urging a "national assault" on disparities.

This seemed truly monumental—an "accelerated national assault" on disparities, called for, not by Black institutions, but by
the government itself, with all the weight and credibility of the
government's health establishment behind it. Whatever frustration and sense of disregard Sullivan, Satcher, and their colleagues
may have felt during their long wait now washed away in a
moment.

When they met with Heckler after learning that the task force
had completed its work, Heckler mentioned that her endodontist
back in Boston was Black. The moment she said that, Rueben Warren, the dean of Meharry School of Dentistry and one of the
AMHPS leaders, cut in. "Yes, I can tell you exactly who that is.
Dr. Bill Walker. He's a professor at the Boston University School
of Dentistry. I know him well. He's the only Black endodontist
in Boston."

After their get-together, the AMHPS leaders talked about that
brief but telling interchange. Warren's personal connection had
furthered the rapport between themselves and Heckler. It had also
highlighted the scarcity of Black medical professionals. There was
one Black endodontist in Boston, a city with over 120,000 African American residents.

Shortly after the Malone task force submitted their report to her,
Heckler released it to the public as the *Report of the Secretary's Task
Force on Black and Minority Health*, commonly known since then
simply as the Heckler Report. In her letter introducing the report
publicly, Heckler wrote, "[It] signaled a sad and significant fact;
*there was a continuing disparity in the burden of death and illness expe-
rienced by Blacks and other minority Americans*" (emphasis in original). The disparity, she wrote, was "an affront to both to our ideals

and to the ongoing genius of American medicine." The report can and should, she declared, "mark the beginning of the end of the health disparity that has, for so long, cast a shadow on the otherwise splendid American track record of ever improving health."

~

Sullivan, Satcher, Bowie, and Haynes had hoped to make disparities in health care and the shortage of Black health professionals a national issue. The Heckler Report did exactly that and in a more robust way than they ever anticipated. The Secretary's report affirmed and extended the conclusions embodied in their own founding document, which they had put in Heckler's hands when they first met.

The Secretary's report went beyond their expectations in another way as well. The AMHPS paper addressed disparities in Black health and health care. The Heckler Report included Hispanics, Native Americans, and Asian/Pacific Islanders in its detailed examination of inequality. Somewhere along the line, the department had decided to broaden the focus to other groups that were suffering their own disparities. The AMHPS report had triggered in the HHS Department a larger attention to the inequities that marred America's care for its minorities. The Heckler Report itself initiated an awareness of health care disparities that eventually went well beyond Blacks, Hispanics, Native Americans, and Asian/Pacific Islanders to include women, the elderly, gay and lesbian Americans, and other nonmainstream groups with their own histories of disparate care. In that sense the Heckler Report was foundational for the increasing understanding of the distance between America's national ideals and values and the realities of prejudice that erode the possibilities of many minority lives.

The AMHPS study had spoken of the shortened life spans of Black Americans as compared with those of their white compatriots, the higher maternal and infant death rates, and the greater burden of illness. It had focused on the glaring shortage of Black doctors and other health professionals and the role that deficit played in the health crisis faced by African Americans. The Heckler Report, in its 239 pages, also examined in detail the chief illnesses and conditions that led to the mortality and morbidity numbers. Heckler's task force had broken into separate committees that focused on the six leading causes of Black death: cancer; vascular disease; alcohol and drugs; diabetes; homicide, suicide, and accidental injuries; as well as infant mortality. It concluded that minority Americans suffered 60,000 excess deaths each year, that is, deaths over and above what would have been normal if minority health were congruent with mainstream health. Among Black Americans, 42.5 percent of deaths per year would not have happened if Black and white health were on a par with each other.[2] "It was evident," the report declared, "that to bring the health of minorities to the level of all Americans, efforts of monumental proportions were needed."

The report implicitly condemned Reagan funding cutbacks that impacted health care. It termed the disparities in care a "tragic dilemma" and called for "efforts of monumental proportions" necessary to make progress. But rhetoric aside, the report's actual recommendations were far less than monumental. They were mostly directed at possible improvements in the various HHS departments and called for increased public and private awareness of the problems and efforts to counteract them through education and strategies for community involvement and outreach. The report called for better diets, more exercise, better dissemination of health information, and more effective collection and distribution of data on minority health. There was little in it about legislative options to attack the problems it identified so precisely. As a *New York Times* editorial put it, "the devastating findings are followed by limp recommendations."

But despite the anodyne recommendations, in the end the Heckler Report proved to be a transformative force. In subsequent years it precipitated and reinforced significant developments not only in attitudes toward minority health care but in major institutional changes that have realigned perspectives on research and clinical practice and on legislation that has improved health care for millions of Americans.

AMHPS had previously distributed its *Blacks and the Health Professions* report to the members of the Congressional Black Caucus and to other members of Congress who were positioned to change laws and/or support funding. Now they made sure the Heckler Report—a cabinet-level document, not a report generated by an interest group—landed on the appropriate desks. Members of Congress who were focused on health care made use of it in various ways, none more energetically than Louis Stokes, the representative from Ohio who had helped found the Congressional Black Caucus and had created the CBC's Health Brain Trust. Stokes's inner-Cleveland, majority Black district suffered from all the ills that impoverishment exacerbated by racism typically brought with it: deficient schools, high unemployment, high crime rates, inadequate nutrition—a litany of problems highlighted, in his mind, by the suffering due to the glaring lack of decent health care. Health care had always been a leading issue for him, but the Heckler Report, with its detailed account of Black disease and death, transformed Stokes into an impassioned crusader. "I was doing everything I could to help open up the national consciousness about [disparities]," he said. "I wanted mainstream health professionals to understand the gravity of the situation and the level of human suffering it entailed."[3]

Stokes used the power he wielded as a member of the House Appropriations Committee, which regulated expenditures, to move key people towards his goals. When NIH heads of institutes came to the committee for funding, he would say, "You're here asking us to appropriate money for the Institute you're heading. Would you agree that Black Americans have higher rates of heart disease [or cancer or hypertension]? What is your Institute doing to understand this and to address it?" Invariably, the answer would be that the general population studies they were pursuing would help minorities as well as everybody else. But Stokes wouldn't let them off the hook. There were extremely few studies specifically of Blacks (or of Hispanics, or of women), so how disease might affect these groups differently was not only unknown, the subject was hardly on anyone's radar screen. "That is not adequate," Stokes told the directors. "NIH should be looking at these things specifically. Don't you agree?" And in fact they had little choice but to agree.

Stokes had allies in the House—he was a favorite of Speaker Tip O'Neill—and in the Senate, where Ted Kennedy partnered with him in getting legislation passed. Louis Sullivan, David Satcher, and other AMHPS people were members of Stokes's Health Brain Trust, where their thinking and policy recommendations resonated not only with Stokes but with the other Black Caucus members. With AMHPS's own study and now the Heckler Report, AMHPS had laid the groundwork for a legislative assault that was to have enduring consequences.

CHAPTER 6

Landmark Legislation

Margaret Heckler issued the *Report of the Secretary's Task Force on Black and Minority Health* in August 1985. Three months later she was forced out of her position. She'd only had time to take one action in response to the Report's depictions of the dire state of Black health. But that one action was significant. Amidst the pressure she was under to give up her post, she initiated the process that established an Office of Minority Health under a deputy assistant secretary. In doing that, Heckler declared in concrete, institutional terms that the US government had a stake in improving the health of America's minority populations. Despite the platitudes and expressions of concern that occasionally made the news prior to this, Heckler's action was a first.

In retrospect, this was a shot across the bow. Obscure as a deputy assistant secretary's office might have seemed to most people, this was the first official notice that a struggle was underway against disparate health care and the inordinate suffering of disease and death borne by communities of color. (This chapter was written in the middle of the COVID-19 pandemic, which has cast such a harsh spotlight on the persistence of health inequalities.) Up until then, there were no entities or research scientists within the Department of Health and Human Services officially concerned with Black health. Neither the National Institutes of Health (NIH), nor the Centers for Disease Control and Prevention (CDC), nor the Food and Drug Administration (FDA) had a single scientist focused on any aspect of the health of minorities.

The new deputy assistant secretary would be looking at these three organizations and all other HHS-controlled health agencies and facilities. It was the responsibility of the new office to consider minority issues throughout the department and to come up with ideas and proposals to address those issues. There was no research budget attached to the position, but as it turned out, the new office was a precursor to larger developments.

Heckler had no time to respond to or develop her report's recommendations before she found herself out of the secretary's job and on her way to Ireland as the new American ambassador. The official line was that she was a poor administrator, but reports from behind the scenes suggested she was forced out due to pressure from various conservative politicians who believed from the start that Heckler was not sufficiently loyal ideologically. In those quarters Heckler's engagement with minority health care and her apparent intention to examine the socioeconomic issues behind it were not welcome.

As secretary, Heckler had found herself in a hostile environment more or less since her appointment. She had served as a moderate Republican representative for eight terms until she lost her seat to Barney Frank in a surprise defeat, driven by her opposition to abortion. President Reagan had appointed her (after Richard Schweiker's departure) in a demonstration of his willingness to take care of long-standing party stalwarts who had been voted out of office.

But as a moderate on many issues, Heckler didn't fit well with the rightward thrust of the Reagan administration that had come to power in large part through Reagan's Southern strategy appeal to white voters. Heckler's issues were not their issues, and HHS, the repository of welfare programs, Medicare/Medicaid, and Social Security, was not an administration priority. Few of Reagan's appointees and advisors cared much about either HHS or Heckler, and Don Regan, the president's powerful chief of staff, personally disliked her. Those circumstances made her embrace of minority health care a distinctive and forthright undertaking. In the long view, the *Report of the Secretary's Task Force on Black and Minority Health* was the signature achievement of Margaret Heckler's political life.

The meeting with AMHPS had precipitated the Heckler Report. The AMHPS white paper, too, was a signature achievement and had been the product of close cooperation among the Black institutional leaders as they defined their priorities and determined the most effective ways to approach legislators and policy makers. Led by school presidents Louis Sullivan and David Satcher, Dean Walter Bowie, and Xavier executive vice president Anthony Rachal, the schools had restrained whatever instinct they had to compete for publicly available funds and bound themselves to each other in a common front. The principals understood that what they were doing—this banding together of Black health institutions—was new, even revolutionary. Moreover, theirs were, literally, life and death issues. Militance and energy flowed from that.

The establishment of the deputy assistant secretary of the office of minority health was a potentially breakthrough achievement. At approximately the same time, AMHPS engineered its first legislative accomplishment that actually brought money into school coffers. This was a Title III program administered not by HHS but by the Department of Education. The relevant legislation had originated years before in the creative brain of William ("Bud") Blakey, Illinois senator Paul Simon's chief of staff.

Bud Blakey was the first African American chief of staff to a US senator. Working closely with Simon, a leading proponent of higher education, Blakey was adept at formulating and writing position papers and crafting legislation. In 1978 Morehouse School of Medicine was still in its start-up period, and in casting around for funding sources, Sullivan had met with Blakey to discuss possibilities. Sullivan explained Morehouse's situation regarding its recent assurance of provisional accreditation and its commitment to becoming a four-year rather than a two-year school. (At that time two-year medical schools were not uncommon; Dartmouth College, the University of Nevada, and the University of North Dakota were two-year schools. Students would do their preclinical science studies at a two-year school, then transfer to a four-year school to finish their degrees.) Blakey thought he could see a way to generate government funding that would be specifically earmarked for Morehouse. Blakey was so enthusiastic about the emergence of what was the first Black medical school in a hundred years that he worked nonstop on his own time to draft an amendment to the Title III Higher Education Act that was coming up soon for reauthorization.

At that time Part B of Title III provided funding for undergraduate institutions. Blakey's amendment proposed an addition, Section 326, that stipulated funding for graduate institutions as well, specifically for two-year medical schools that had received provisional accreditation and were committed to expanding to four-year programs. His amendment included other defining criteria and specified that the funding was for "historically Black" institutions. Only one institution in the country qualified under the Blakey amendment: Morehouse School of Medicine.

The Georgia congressional delegation worked on the bill alongside Sullivan and Blakey. Congressman Lou Stokes from Ohio shepherded it through the House. When the Senate changed to Republican control, Arlen Specter sponsored it there, with support from the chair of the Senate Appropriations Committee, Mark Hatfield. The bill passed, giving Morehouse School of Medicine enough funding to build its first building and to start getting out of the rental and trailer space it occupied at Morehouse College. This was a remarkable piece of enabling legislation, remarkable too that it passed with little scrutiny and no opposition, which speaks to the political heft behind it. In the Carter administration (1977–1981) both chambers were under Democratic control, and the spirit of Lyndon Johnson's Great Society had not yet been extinguished. In some ways that spirit kept a tenuous hold on life even after Ronald Reagan was elected.

The Section 326 provision became law in 1978, although it wasn't funded until 1981. Eight years later, with the Heckler Report behind them and another Title III reauthorization coming up, the AMHPS board began discussing whether or not the association's other schools might be folded into eligibility. The additional funding would be meaningful, and among themselves—Sullivan, Satcher, Bowie, and the others—worked out a formula by which a few schools at a time would qualify for inclusion. They didn't want to try to include too many at once so that the provision would stay beneath the radar and pass more or less automatically. As a result, the criteria for inclusion were successfully amended, and Meharry, Charles Drew, and Tuskegee soon became eligible for funding.

In succeeding years, the other AMHPS schools were folded in, then other historically Black schools that were not AMHPS members. Since the first amendment in 1978, Section 326 has been reauthorized various times and the criteria amended further. In

2020 (at the time of this writing), eighteen institutions are included in this Act to Strengthen Historically Black Graduate Institutions that prepare students "in the legal, medical, dental, veterinary, math, engineering and physical and natural science fields." Bud Blakey's original amendment, meant only for Morehouse School of Medicine, has evolved over forty years into a significant catalyst and core funding for many institutions across many disciplines.

~

In concert, the AMHPS institutions were finding ways to strengthen themselves, this in a culture where Black schools; Black physicians, dentists and pharmacists; and most importantly, the health of Black Americans had historically been under great duress. But the pressures felt by the AMHPS schools were internal as well as external. Morehouse School of Medicine had originated the Title III program when AMHPS was in its early years. Now the other institutions were eager to join and become eligible for funding as well. In the conferences about this, a "hold harmless" solution was formulated that insured that Morehouse, which had conceptualized the program and developed the legislation for it, would not suffer financially. Whatever funding might become available through Title III for additional institutions, the Morehouse distribution would not be affected. In addition, since it wasn't feasible to bring in all the other schools at once, they had to find agreement on the order in which more schools would be included. With funding at stake, these were potentially divisive problems, the kind that would have severely strained any coalition. But the presidents and deans were able to temper their differences and see their way through the conflicts. It was, in Sullivan's words, "a remarkable period of cooperation and mutual support."

It was only a few years, though, before AMHPS's all-for-one-and-one-for-all spirit was tested almost to the breaking point. The "hold harmless" provision in the principals' agreement meant that the new schools that came aboard after Morehouse needed to advocate for additional funding to build the Section 326 pool. That went well as Meharry, Charles Drew, and Tuskegee were folded in as the first cohort of additional schools. But by the time the next opportunity for more schools to join came up, federal funding had tightened. Believing it would be difficult to procure additional funds, Florida A&M president, Frederick Humphries, pressed the AMHPS board to drop the hold harmless provision so that Florida A&M College of Pharmacy would share in funds, even if the overall funding was not increased. Beyond that, he believed that since Morehouse had been benefitting from this legislation for a number of years, they should drop out of the program altogether and leave the entire pool of money to the other schools.

This did not sit well with Sullivan, who, along with Bud Blakey, had written the legislation for the benefit of Morehouse and had then agreed to expand it as a funding platform for the other AMHPS schools. AMHPS board meetings, which had always been congenial and mutually supportive, grew tense and adversarial. In the middle of the controversy, it became known that Humphries was meeting with key members of the House Education Committee, demanding the changes he wanted regardless of the AMHPS internal agreement.

As the conflict flared, William Clay, who had partnered with Lou Stokes in founding the Congressional Black Caucus, stepped in, calling a meeting with Humphries, Sullivan, and a few other AMHPS leaders. In blunt terms, Clay and Stokes told the leaders that what was going on was not tolerable, that they were in danger of cutting off their nose to spite their face. Not only was this controversy likely to destroy the legislation altogether, which they—Clay and Stokes—had worked so hard to put in place, but it would affect their credibility on the Hill. The two congressmen told them, in effect, to leave this conflict alone and get back to working for their mutual benefit.

When it was clear which way the wind was blowing, President Humphries backed off. In the end, the next cohort of schools, including Florida A&M, were folded in, and Section 326 went on, gathering more schools under its aegis as it went. But it had been a close call.

~

AMHPS chief lobbyist Harley Dirks (Senator Warren Magnuson's former Appropriations Committee staff director) had shepherded the association through its early period. But in 1985 Harley retired, and his son Dale replaced him. Dale Dirks's approach to institutional support was focused on law-based funding specifically geared toward the AMHPS schools. The alternative was competitive grants, which were problematic. Grants were awarded and sustained, or not, through a competitive process. They were time limited; and sustaining them was always precarious. But law-based funding was embedded in statute. It did not typically go away but continued as a stable stream of support. The level of funding had to be argued for in the yearly federal budgeting process, so amounts might go up or down, but the funding source itself stayed in place. Law-based funding became a legacy that could support expansion beyond the original institutions it was written for. AMHPS Title III funding—Strengthening Historically Black Graduate Institutions—fit that description. So did AMHPS's next big achievement: Title VII legislation—the Excellence in Minority Health Education and Care Act.

The idea for the Excellence in Minority Health Education and Care Act originated with David Satcher. Satcher had become president of Meharry Medical College in 1982, at a time when Meharry was in such desperate financial straits that it seemed the school's more-than-one-hundred-year history was drawing quickly to a close. Satcher put reforms in place that had rescued the school from an immediate demise, but five years later Meharry was still skating near the edge.

Meharry Medical College and Meharry Dental School were receiving small grants each year through the Advanced Financial Distress Program that had been established as part of the Public Health Service Act. Xavier University College of Pharmacy and Tuskegee School of Veterinary Medicine were also in the program. The funding authority made these grants available to distressed institutions to help meet debt commitments and to address accreditation requirements, but they didn't deal with the many other needs that pressed on these old-line Black institutions. Moreover, in 1987 the law would soon be reaching its mandated expiration date.

These four schools had been leaders in training Black physicians, pharmacists, dentists, and veterinarians for many decades, two had been training leaders for more than a century. But with the vast bulk of their students coming from impoverished, often rural backgrounds, they had never built more than threadbare endowments, which meant their endowments didn't have the wherewithal to see the schools through particularly stressful times. Unlike the Harvards or Columbias of the medical world, their graduates commonly established primary practices in rural areas and filled essential roles in severely underserved communities; very few went on to do the kind of research and achieve the medical science breakthroughs that generated attention and attracted large gifts to better-known institutions.

David Satcher came from a family of ten children in the farming region near Anniston, Alabama, a place where few Black children ever finished high school, much less went to college. But

Satcher's parents had recognized his talents and kept him out of the fields long enough for him to concentrate on studying. They might have been subsistence farmers, but they put a high value on education; and they were not the kind of people who just accepted their lot and were content with thinking, okay, that's just the way things are.

Satcher inherited his parents' spirit. He attended Morehouse College on a scholarship, but unlike the many Morehouse premedical students who went on to Meharry or Howard, he aimed toward one of the prestigious Northern institutions and was accepted at Case Western in Cleveland, Ohio, where he earned a medical degree and simultaneously a PhD in cell biology.

Twelve years later Satcher came to Meharry as president from an already distinguished career in medical science. He had been director of the King/Drew Medical Center Sickle Cell Research Center and a professor at UCLA. But under financial pressures as president of Meharry, he got to thinking that the contribution his school had made in terms of training doctors to serve in some of the nation's most badly neglected places was no less important than the achievements of great research institutions like Harvard, Columbia, or Johns Hopkins in fighting cancer and other major diseases. Meharry, he thought, ought to be recognized and rewarded for its immense, historic contribution to public health. And not just Meharry Medical College, but Meharry Dental, Xavier University College of Pharmacy, and Tuskegee School of Veterinary Medicine, the other old-line Black institutions receiving distressed financial aid funding—now running out for all of them.

The role they played, he thought, should be recognized through funding legislation, but he had never liked the connotation of the Financial Distress Program. Meharry and its sister schools were poor and distressed, but they shouldn't be denigrated as institutional beggars. They most definitely should not regard themselves or portray themselves that way. They should be lauded because of what they'd done for health care in the nation's most needy places, which they did better than anyone else could. Considering the obstacles they had faced throughout their history, their contribution to the nation's health was in reality nothing less than heroic.

Thinking along these lines, Satcher and Dale Dirks began sketching out legislation they believed would appropriately recognize Meharry and the others. Together with Tuskegee's Walter Bowie and Xavier's Marcellus Grace (dean of the pharmacy school and an AMHPS board member), they gave concrete form to a program they named the Excellence in Minority Health Education and Care Act, an amendment to Title VII of the Public Health Service Act. From the start, they thought that if they could get it passed, they could then expand it to build the funding levels and include the other AMHPS institutions, using the same "hold harmless" mechanism they had used for expansion of the Title III Strengthening Historically Black Graduate Institutions Act.

The question was, Could they get it passed?

Xavier was in Louisiana, Tuskegee in Alabama, Meharry in Tennessee. These institutions were all fixtures in their states. Tuskegee School of Veterinary Medicine was part of Tuskegee University, founded in 1881 by Booker T. Washington and later home to the great agricultural scientist George Washington Carver, as well as to the Tuskegee Airmen, the Black fighter groups that fought in World War II. Its veterinary school was the only predominantly African American school of its kind in the country. Tuskegee had considerable support in Alabama. Likewise, Meharry had serious support in Tennessee, especially from Nashville-area legislators. Meharry was the second Black medical school in the country; its history went back to 1876. Meharry, too, had white as well as Black supporters, proud that this historic institution was located in their home place. Xavier University was not just a Black fixture in New Orleans; it was a Catholic institution, founded by Saint Katharine Drexel and the Sisters of the Blessed Sacrament. Xavier University president, Norman Francis, was a thought leader on education in Louisiana in both the Black and white communities, was highly regarded by Senator J. Bennett Johnston, and was important for his influence among Black voters. Johnston, like all Louisiana politicians, was extremely parochial when it came to the state's educational institutions. Xavier's financial stability was important on many counts to people who mattered in Louisiana.

The four schools had important constituencies, which carried a good deal of weight as Dale Dirks made the rounds of the Alabama, Tennessee, and Louisiana congressional delegations to gather support for the Excellence in Minority Health amendment. Louisiana's Johnston agreed to sponsor the bill in the Senate, and he brought along Ted Kennedy and other Senate power brokers. The markup went through committee easily and passed the Senate with bipartisan support.

The House process was dicier. There, Congressman Bill Boner from Nashville took the lead. Boner had always been a strong supporter of Meharry, so he was happy to sponsor the bill. But as hearings were about to start in Henry Waxman's subcommittee on health and the environment, Boner became embroiled in an ethics probe, serious enough that it threatened his tenure. As the ethics investigation gathered steam, Boner went to Waxman and told him that he was probably going to have to resign. Would Waxman please, he asked, consider this bill before he needed to do that.

Waxman agreed and put it on his committee's agenda for immediate action. At that time, the House allowed proxy voting, which meant that in situations where a quorum wasn't present, the committee chair and the ranking member were considered to hold the proxy votes of their party members. The chairperson could call the meeting to order, and as long as the ranking member was present, the committee could proceed to a vote. In that situation, the only recourse the ranking member had was to object to the absence of a quorum.

On the given day, Waxman banged his gavel and called the meeting to order. Only Waxman and the ranking member, William Dannemeyer, were present. Dannemeyer was an archconservative Republican from California's Orange County who had, among other actions, vigorously opposed gay rights and attempted to block funding for the Smithsonian's exhibits on evolution. He regularly voted to cut budgets for social programs. The Excellence in Minority Health Education and Care Act was exactly the kind of bill that made him see red. Dannemeyer's nickname among his House colleagues was "Dynamiter." He was a tough nut; Waxman later described him as "a mean and hateful person."

When Waxman called the meeting to order and introduced the bill, Dannemeyer wasted no time declaring his objection, which meant consideration of the bill was dead, at least for that session. That was a problem. Waxman wasn't happy about not being able to proceed. He didn't like that kind of failure happening in his committee. He knew that the committee members all had different work going on in their other committee assignments and for their constituents, and that a single agenda item like this could well go unattended. Meanwhile, Dannemeyer had objected once. If Waxman brought it up again, Dannemeyer's response would be exactly the same. "This is going to be a waste of my time," Waxman told Dale Dirks.

Dirks and his colleagues were scrambling. Since the Tennessee delegation was on board, they went to Tennessee Republican Congressman Jimmy Quillen, telling him that the legislation he had cosponsored had been knocked down by Dannemeyer. Quillen, a twelve-term representative, was part of the Republican leadership, a hard man for fellow Republicans to say no to. But Dannemeyer was an inveterate obstructionist, adamant in his opposition to initiatives he didn't like, and this was one he really didn't like.

After talking with Dirks, Quillen found Dannemeyer on the floor of the House. "Listen," he said, "I want that bill to go through, with no quorum objections." Dannemeyer listened, but he made no commitments, which is what Dirks went back to Waxman with. "We don't know what he'll do," Dirks said, "but we do know he received the message."

The following week Waxman reconvened the subcommittee. Again the only members present were himself and Dannemayer, along with seven or eight staff onlookers. Their eyes were fixed on Dannemeyer, who sat there stone-faced as Waxman banged his gavel and called the session to order. "The committee will now consider the Excellence in Minority Education and Care Act." He waited. "Are there any objections?" Dannemeyer's expression was grim, but he kept his mouth shut, obviously with great effort. He did not object. With that, the bill sailed out of subcommittee and was approved by the House, again with bipartisan support.

Two years later, AMHPS and AMHPS's chief congressional sponsor, Lou Stokes, amended the Excellence in Minority Health Education and Care Act to fold in the other AMHPS institutions, again with a similar "hold harmless" feature that protected the funding of the original four schools. At that point AMHPS was approached by several Hispanic-serving institutions and Native American–serving institutions requesting that they too might be included under the act. There was some arguing back and forth with them about the hold harmless provision, although nothing like the turbulence that had roiled the AMHPS schools earlier.

With no objections from AMHPS, the other minority-serving institutions were also included.

AMHPS's original white paper was an effort by Black institutions to draw attention to Black health and the pressing need for more Black medical professionals. The Heckler Report, which the AMHPS paper precipitated, addressed the health and disparities of other minorities as well. A similar process took place here too. An act initiated by and intended for Black institutions expanded its scope to include other minorities. The AMHPS leaders were focused on their own institutions and communities; they were not thinking of the overarching problem of inequalities in the health care of minorities generally. But the dynamic had its own momentum. Opening an argument for the needs and rights of one dispossessed group seemed by its nature to broaden attention to other groups suffering their own inequities, inevitable perhaps in a system where equality is a primary value, no matter how deficient in the observance.

Among other purposes, the Excellence in Minority Health Education and Care Act was meant to "establish, strengthen, or expand programs to increase the number and quality of applicants for admission." In that regard it was a landmark, the first government program that specifically recognized the need to increase the numbers of minority health professionals, AMHPS's primary motive, defined so memorably in the 1983 white paper. In including Hispanic and Native American institutions, the act also solidified political support by engaging a broader array of legislators, a principle that first revealed its strategic benefits when Morehouse and Mercer medical schools became allies in the fight for capitation funding in the Georgia legislature more than a decade earlier.

~

Over the years some of the AMHPS leaders had developed contacts within NIH, often having to do with research or clinical matters at their institutions. That was how Sullivan had gotten to know William Raub, who in the mid-1980s was NIH's deputy director. Prior to that, Raub had been deputy director for extramural research, which meant that he oversaw grants to scientists at outside institutions, including grants sought by Morehouse medical school investigators.

Morehouse, like other Black institutions, had a spotty record when it came to winning NIH grant awards. With that in mind, Sullivan started a discussion with Raub about the need Morehouse had to strengthen its science research and the disadvantage his school and others were at in this very competitive arena. The priority for Morehouse and the other AMHPS schools was preparing front-line clinicians, yet research was also significant for them, especially given the absence of any national effort to understand the specific disease profile of African Americans or the impact of the stark health care disparities they suffered from.

Raub listened carefully to Sullivan and found himself agreeing with the desirability of building up research capability at Morehouse and other AMHPS schools. He noted that some years earlier NIH had established a program to support research in states that didn't have the great medical science infrastructure of places like New York, California, or Massachusetts. The idea of strengthening Morehouse and other Black institutions was consistent with that; moreover the rationale, he thought, was persuasive and timely.

Once Sullivan and Raub had sketched out how this might be done, they took the idea to Louis Stokes, who for years now had been pressing his congressional colleagues to recognize and address the dire circumstances of minority health. Stokes himself had grown up in Cleveland's projects. He had worked his way through law school at night and had become a sought-after criminal defense lawyer and head of Cleveland's NAACP Legal Redress Committee. His younger brother, Carl, was the country's first Black mayor of a major city, while Stokes was Ohio's first ever Black congressman. As much as anyone, the two Stokes brothers had carved out a place in the nation's political life for the recognition of Black participation and Black legislative power. "I'm here," President Obama had told Stokes, "because of you and your brother."

From the start of Louis Stokes's long congressional tenure, the health of his community had been forefront in his mind. Stokes embraced Raub and Sullivan's approach, as they knew he would. With help from AMHPS, he and his staff put together a bill that mandated funding for equipment such as centrifuges and electron microscopes, for technicians and other laboratory staff, and for support for principal investigators. The intention was to build up the science research capability of the AMHPS schools, not just to enable them to compete better but to bring focused research to bear on diseases that disproportionately affected minority populations, a nearly wholly neglected backwater in research on public health.

They titled the bill the Research Centers in Minority Institutions (RCMI) Program. Louis Stokes had by now achieved even greater leverage than he had previously. He had chaired the Select Committee on the Assassinations of Martin Luther King and John F. Kennedy. He had chaired the House Ethics Committee. He was a senior member of the Appropriations Committee and was on his way to assuming the chair of an appropriations subcommittee, which was to give him control of large sums of the federal budget. He was known for his probity and evenhandedness, trusted even by his political opponents. Armed with statistics and arguments furnished by AMHPS and his own staff, and waving the Heckler Report in front of skeptics, Stokes was an effective, forceful advocate. The bill met little opposition in the House and was incorporated into the 1986 appropriations act for HHS and related agencies. It was not part of the corresponding Senate appropriations bill, but the House/Senate conference committee accepted the House version, which became law in 1986. With the law's passage, RCMI became an HHS responsibility, administered under NIH's National Center for Research Resources.

In the course of its adoption there were few dissenters in Congress. Racial politics played no discernible role—among appropriators it was embraced on both sides of the aisle. But RCMI was the first AMHPS effort that involved NIH, and at NIH there was a swell of institutional unhappiness, despite William Raub's role. NIH was informed by a competitive, peer review culture. The Institutes were instinctively unreceptive to mandates that laid down what their course of action needed to be, particularly when it concerned the issuing of grants.

NIH's director, Dr. James Wyngaarden, was a highly regarded scientist and administrator. He was also a firm believer in the peer review model. For him and many others at the Institutes, strong peer-reviewed grant applications were what needed to drive the decision-making process, not mandates regarding infrastructure and the development of new programs that opened pathways outside the ingrained culture. As a result, although nobody could reasonably argue that health disparities were unimportant, there was significant pushback within the Institutes. This didn't fade over time. In troubling ways it became an abrasive factor as NIH was drawn further into engagement with minority health issues.

～

The AMHPS leaders presented their case to Secretary Heckler in the spring of 1983. She in turn issued the *Report of the Secretary's Task Force on Black and Minority Health* in August 1985. The following two years saw landmark legislation that brought the government face-to-face with the reality of health disparities and the massive, disproportionate amount of disease and excessive deaths that were its consequence. In each of these cases, AMHPS drove the legislative process.

In the course of these few years, the groundwork was laid for ongoing decades of engagement, hope, accomplishment, frustration, and anger that have characterized America's attempts to address the health inequities that afflict its minority communities. African American health institutions had witnessed the power of concerted action, and they were able to develop meaningful support from lawmakers across party lines. They succeeded in strengthening themselves financially, building up infrastructure and research capabilities, and improving their admissions reach. These had a cumulative effect, not just for the institutions themselves but for the awakening recognition among lawmakers of the national crisis—and disgrace—represented by disparate health care. In these years AMHPS charted the waters. The association acquired an awareness of what worked, what didn't, what the dangers were, and something about the headwinds that might be in the offing.

CHAPTER 7

AMHPS
and the Secretary

The productivity of the years 1986 through 1988 was driven by AMHPS and the commitment of many in Congress, especially Louis Stokes. Stokes was a force to be reckoned with, but the legislation—Strengthening Black Graduate Institutions, Excellence in Minority Health Education, and Research Centers at Minority Institutions—received support from Republicans as well as Democrats. That wasn't an accident. From the beginning AMHPS had pursued a bipartisan strategy.

The organization had come into being during the Carter years. Then in 1980 Ronald Reagan was elected president, and his first budget slashed education expenditures, which had a devastating impact on Black medical school students, many of who depended on the now eviscerated National Health Service Corps scholarship program. But the AMHPS leadership knew that political winds shift and that their issues needed support regardless of which party was in power. As a result, all through the 1980s they worked to cultivate contacts and friends on both sides of the aisle; it was a deliberate strategy. They had courted Secretary Heckler in 1983, and for their landmark bills they lobbied Republicans as hard as they lobbied Democrats. Generally, they found Republicans supportive, some of them enthusiastically so. Republicans Arlen Specter, Mark Hatfield, and Robert Packwood took lead roles at different times. Silvio Conte from Massachusetts was another staunch Republican ally.

Conte was the ranking member of the House Appropriations Committee during the Reagan years, a colleague of Louis Stokes. Stokes regularly argued for money to fund the minority health bills, which he did vigorously but also with some discomfort. Stokes was the single Black member of the committee, and he felt awkward pressing for Black health bills in front of a committee full of white members. That was awkward, not that it ever deflected him from what he was doing, but the awkwardness bothered him. "I did what I thought I had to do," he wrote later. "That went on for years, during a great deal of my tenure on one or another of the Appropriations committees, twenty-eight out of my thirty years in Congress altogether. It was not comfortable for me, and it was not comfortable for those sitting there on the hot seat answering question after question from this Black man about Black people—at a time and in a context where they weren't thinking much about Black people at all."[1]

Conte understood the awkwardness of Stokes's situation, and he sometimes put himself in the middle. Others did also, taking Stokes's list of questions and presenting them for him. At one point when the Democratic chair, William Natcher, thought Stokes's request for funds was excessive, Conte came and sat down next to Stokes. "How much will you take on this?" Conte whispered. Stokes told him. A short time later Conte said, "Mr. Chairman, I think we ought to fund it at this rate."

"What was the chairman going to do then?" Stokes recalled later. "He wasn't going to oppose his ranking member. "All right, all right," Natcher said. "I guess we'll have to put that number in."[2]

Republican support was, if anything, a priority. Democrats were more instinctively favorable to these bills, so AMHPS devoted considerable effort to Republicans. Their support was always helpful; on occasion it was critical. When the initial Title III appropriations bill was up for reconciliation between the House and Senate versions, Democrat Senator David Boren moved to strip out all special funding measures from the omnibus spending bill, which would have eliminated the Morehouse School of Medicine's Section 326 amendment that Bud Blakey and Sullivan had worked so hard on—which would have relegated the funding of Black institutions funding to nothing.

By then Republican Mack Mattingly had defeated Democrat Herman Talmadge for one of Georgia's senate seats (Mattingly was the first Republican senator elected in the state since Reconstruction). Mattingly was hard core; he had chaired Barry Goldwater's campaign in Georgia. At the same time he was a Morehouse medical school supporter. Mattingly recruited Mississippi Republican Senator Thad Cochran, and together they successfully filibustered Boren's motion, which saved Morehouse's funding and made possible the later AMHPS funding. Two Republicans, in other words, joined together to defeat a Democrat on an issue of fundamental importance to Black professional and graduate schools.

The Reagan congresses of the middle 1980s were often fierce political battlegrounds. With Democrats controlling the House, and Republicans the Senate, and with a popular conservative president, fiscal debates were especially heated. But minority health care issues often sidestepped the warfare. In fact, Black health

institutions found themselves in a social and political environment that hadn't existed in the hundred plus years since Reconstruction. In the post–World War II years, America had been
coming to grips with the exclusion of African Americans from full
citizenship. The civil rights movement, hard fought and often
bloody, had shifted the nation's mindset on the matter of equality. Martin Luther King's assassination had jolted that shift up a
notch. The national discussions triggered by school integration,
voting rights legislation, and employment and fair housing legislation had led to changes of perception among many mainstream
Americans regarding the justice of Black efforts to achieve equality. Since the Kennedy, Johnson, and Nixon administrations,
"affirmative action" had become embedded as a national strategy to advance inclusion.

The changed atmosphere was marked not just by a shift in white
perceptions but by a newly robust mobilization of resources within
the Black community. In the judicial world, Thurgood Marshall's
elevation to the Supreme Court had injected a new viewpoint into
high-level legal proceedings, which sifted down to considerations
in lower courts. Even justices who may not have agreed with Marshall's views now found it necessary to take his perspective into
account. In Congress, the 1968 general election had raised the
number of Black representatives to nine, a watershed. Nine Black
representatives had never before served together in the House,
even during Reconstruction. Shortly after taking office, Louis
Stokes and William Clay had organized what became the Congressional Black Caucus—an independent, Black political power
bloc—an altogether novel element on the American political
scene. "The stage had been set," Stokes wrote later, "for an asser-
tive emergence of black political power."[3]

At the same time, the Ford Foundation helped fund a
Washington-based think tank focused on Black issues, the Joint

Center for Political and Economic Studies, another first. By the mid-1980s the CBC's nine members had grown to twenty, a number of who were by then climbing the ladder of seniority on various committees. Black Americans had never before played a role in national politics. Now they had not only carved out space, they were expanding their presence.

AMHPS had come to life as a specific answer to the needs of the Black health professions institutions. But from a historical perspective, it was part of a wave of births that represented the mustering of Black strength during a time of optimism and hope. The legislative successes of 1985, 1986, and 1987 benefited from a broad national sense that racial inequalities needed to be addressed and ameliorated, not least in terms of health care. Margaret Heckler had written in her release of the *Report of the Secretary's Task Force on Black and Minority Health* that she hoped the report would signal the beginning of the end of health disparities. Sullivan, Satcher, Bowie, Rachal, and the other AMHPS leaders knew what a daunting objective that was, but they thought that they were, at last, making a good start. "Now, Sullivan said, "we had the power to really work in order to do something about it. Not to depend on others but to take the initiative in addressing these issues ourselves."

AMHPS made its entrance onto the national stage in 1985. It was then that the association began its full-fledged engagement with the legislative process. At the same time the member schools—Meharry, Tuskegee, Xavier, Morehouse, Florida A&M, Texas Southern, and Charles Drew—were learning each other's cultures and management styles. They were figuring out how to more effectively network with each other and how best to leverage each other's political strengths.

The AMHPS member schools called seven states home, which meant that seven cohorts of Congressional representatives were possible, perhaps likely, supporters. In addition, the Congressional

Black Caucus now included representatives from a considerable number of states. In some places, African American state legislators had formed their own Black caucuses. Only a few years earlier, AMHPS's leaders were casting around for how they might bring their issues into national awareness and how to attract legislative attention. They had now found their way; already they were growing adept at using the levers of power.

As if to mark the association's transition from a self-contained coalition to a national catalyst on minority health issues, AMHPS's presidency now rotated from Sullivan to Tuskegee's Walter Bowie. From the beginning the concept had been to rotate leadership from one institution to another. Sullivan had seen that principle at work in the Atlanta University Center Consortium made up of Atlanta University and Morehouse, Spelman, Clark, and Morris Brown colleges, which gave each institution a rotating leadership role and concretized the idea of equality among the schools. AMHPS founders had built that same principle into the association's governance. They considered rotation a binding element in an organization where there was a natural, ongoing tension between the self-interest of its member institutions and the cohesion necessary for their continued success.

Sullivan had founded the organization and steered it through its maturation and its entrance onto the national scene. The legislative accomplishments that followed during Walter Bowie's tenure were, in effect, pieces of a puzzle. The Title III funding went toward strengthening the institutions generally; Title VII funding toward stimulating enrollment and enhancing teaching resources; RCMI toward building research capability. But while these successes created a powerful sense of optimism, all the leaders recognized that developing their new strengths was going to take time. None of their institutions had previously received this level of federal support. All of them—the older ones like Meharry and

Tuskegee, and the new ones like Morehouse and Charles Drew—
were at the starting line of development.

On the congressional front, the work to create and pass the
three pieces of legislation had absorbed much of the association's
energy and resources. Now the association and Dale Dirks, its
lobbyist, turned their attention to the business of getting and
keeping the legislation funded. Passing federal legislation that
acknowledged and addressed the health care needs of America's
minorities was historic. But the laws themselves meant nothing
unless their provisions were funded. As a result, the association's
efforts shifted from the authorizing committees to the appropriating committees. The legislation had been enacted; now came
the business of persuading the appropriating committees to fund
them at adequate levels. Presidents Bowie and Satcher, along with
Marcellus Grace, dean of the Xavier University College of Pharmacy, took the lead in working with the House and Senate Appropriations Committees in what proved to be an arduous process.

While the legislation itself had been passed with bipartisan support, the Reagan budgets were austere, reversing the previous
trend by cutting expenditures on social welfare programs while increasing allocations for the military. In that environment the challenge for AMHPS and its supporters was figuring out how to
extract money from a shrinking pool of available funds. Making
sure that these three new and important programs received adequate support through the annual appropriations process was, in
Dirks's words, "a handful."

~

Each of the three AMHPS-initiated acts of 1986 and 1987 contributed to the strength of the association's institutions. But the Research Centers in Minority Institutions (RCMI) Act also looked
specifically at building the AMHPS schools' ability to address the
overarching problem of disparate, inferior health care. RCMI

provided funding for research infrastructure that would help the schools attract high level medical scientists and compete for research grants. Those new resources would, the leaders expected, give their schools the wherewithal to begin studying the spectrum of disease patterns and specific health disabilities facing African Americans.

All the AMHPS institutions were eligible for this funding, as were other minority-serving schools that offered PhDs, sixteen schools in all. But the initial funding was only $4.7 million, which meant grant applications were going to be scrutinized with extreme care. The NIH manager responsible for this was Sidney McNairy, a former biochemistry professor at Southern University, a historically Black institution in Louisiana. In 1986 McNairy had been at NIH for over a decade. He had come originally with the objective of learning how Southern University could write more-effective grant applications. NIH's standard "RO1" research grants were highly competitive, minutely judged by committees of experts. To be successful, an application needed to be elegant, sophisticated, and focused. The proposed research needed to address fundamental problems. It needed to access relevant institutional support. RO1 grants were a world unto themselves, a world the AMHPS schools and other historically Black institutions had little experience with. McNairy had thought to stay only a year. But NIH had offered him a full-time job and he had accepted.

McNairy, an African American, was a dynamic, adept administrator with a strong creative streak. The RCMI program gave him an opportunity to devote his talents to helping institutions high on his list of priorities. When the legislation passed, he visited all sixteen eligible schools, not only to assess their ability to utilize funding but to look at what kind of funding might make the biggest impact.

RCMI's stated objective was "to enhance the research environment at minority colleges and universities in the health sciences." McNairy concluded that the grants he was awarding and administering should be regarded strategically, not just to enhance the research environment but to give the recipient institutions the ability to attract what he thought of as "magnet investigators." He saw that schools with superstar health scientists benefited widely from their presence. Nobel laureates and other breakthrough scientists not only won grants themselves, they fed the reputation of their home institutions, attracting high-level colleagues and top students, and modeling or pointing out potentially fruitful directions for research.

Research infrastructure, he thought, should be configured to attract that level of investigator. Black health institutions, with their traditional grass-roots orientation, could boast few of these medical science luminaries. McNairy set out to change that. "My goal," he said, "was to put these institutions in a position where they could recruit top African American scientists."[4]

With McNairy's help, Meharry was able to construct a CDC-classified Biosafety Level 3 laboratory, which enabled research on microbes that cause serious and potentially lethal disease, such as tuberculosis, Eastern equine encephalitis, yellow fever, and bubonic plague. At Howard (which joined AMHPS in 1994), RCMI funding bought sophisticated equipment, FACS (fluorescence-activated cell sorting) machines, essential to isolating and studying living cells. Next-generation electron microscopes were also on McNairy's shopping list. RCMI helped Morehouse and Tuskegee acquire these. McNairy also persuaded the Pacific Northwest National Laboratory to provide CAGE (computer assisted generative engineering) machines for gene sequencing, which he set up in six centers around the country, enabling a high level of collaborative research among the AMHPS schools. Several AMHPS institutions expanded animal research laboratories and facilities to care for and maintain the animals.

Over time, the upgrade in their research environments did attract some of the nation's top scientists, just as McNairy hoped it would. Garry Gibbons, a leading research cardiologist, went from Harvard to Morehouse School of Medicine, where he founded the Cardiovascular Research Institute. James Hildreth, a Rhodes scholar specializing in immunology, left a professorship at Johns Hopkins to go to Meharry Medical College, where he did groundbreaking research on AIDS. Morehouse recruited Peter MacLeish from the Rockefeller Institute and Cornell. At his new home MacLeish founded the Morehouse Neuroscience Institute. Keith Norris, a nephrologist at Drew, and James Townsel, a neuroscientist at Meharry, were also leaders in their fields. When he first arrived at Meharry (from Harvard), Townsel was the only neuroscientist at the school. RCMI funding enabled him to hire five additional researchers and teachers in his field. Over the years he trained eight African American neuroscience PhDs.

When the RCMI program was established, none of the AMHPS faculties included a member of the National Academy of Science. By the time Sidney McNairy retired from his position, every one of them did.

McNairy's magnet investigators played the role he had envisioned, from putting the AMHPS schools on the map in terms of grant proposals to attracting high-level colleagues eager to work with them. The names and the upgraded lab facilities made the schools more attractive when it came to recruiting faculty. Prospective faculty members in the medical sciences were now more attracted to these institutions that were prepared to foster their research, where they wouldn't be overwhelmed by teaching

responsibilities in service to the schools' primary mission of training clinicians for work in poor, underserved places.

For many prospective faculty, though, that mission was a
powerful draw, even if they themselves were not primarily clinicians. They liked, and often loved, the idea of being part of a primarily Black institution dedicated not only to educating health
workers but to social justice. They identified strongly with that.
That was something they wanted to be part of, and having a supportive research environment made it easier for them to do it.
They could have stayed where they were or gone on to other
mainstream institutions looking for talented Black faculty, but
affiliating with a Black institution gave an additional sense of
purpose to their lives.

The same was also true for many of the white faculty members
at the AMHPS schools. All the AMHPS schools were predominantly Black institutions; but their faculties were integrated and,
typically, white prospective faculty were also drawn by these
schools' mission and by their own desire to contribute to what they
regarded as a fundamentally important effort.

After the passage of the three AMHPS-initiated acts, the association's energies were largely engaged in the congressional funding effort while the schools themselves began figuring out how
to use the new income streams most effectively. At the same time,
developments at Morehouse School of Medicine presaged an event
that was to have a momentous impact on AMHPS, as it did on the
federal government's engagement with minority health and health
disparities altogether.

～

The origin of this event went back to the original Title III amendment that Bud Blakey had initiated in 1978. Combining the funding from that act together with money raised through its own

fundraising drive, Morehouse School of Medicine had built its first independent building on land the school acquired adjacent to the Morehouse College campus.

The building was scheduled to be completed in December 1981, but construction problems delayed the opening until July 1982. Morehouse president Louis Sullivan had extended an invitation to President Reagan to speak at the dedication ceremony, but the White House response was a long time coming. In the interim, the Reagan budget was passed that cut funding for various domestic programs important to the Black community including, specifically, funds for medical school scholarships for disadvantaged students.

Then came Reagan's support for Bob Jones University's ban on interracial dating. The evangelical school was battling the threatened loss of its tax exemption because of its racially discriminatory practices. But Reagan's Justice Department decided to drop the government's tax case against the school. (The DOJ's action had met with a storm of criticism, and the administration reversed its decision. The university finally lost its battle, and its tax exemption, in 1983.)

"[Reagan's] support for Bob Jones went through the black community like a lead shot," Sullivan wrote later, "which left me thinking what a terrible mistake it had been to invite him."[5] If Reagan did come, Sullivan thought, he'd have to leave town afterwards himself. But how in the world could he possibly disinvite a sitting president?

In the end, Sullivan's dilemma resolved itself. After a four-month delay, the White House responded to his invitation. To Sullivan's vast relief, the answer was "no." Reagan wasn't coming.

But even as Sullivan was breathing a deep sigh of relief, his Washington representative, attorney Ray Cotton, told him that since Reagan wasn't coming, he should try to get Vice President

George H. W. Bush. "It's important for you to develop these relationships," Cotton said. "You can write to the White House how
disappointed you are. . . . Perhaps in light of the circumstances the
vice president might be able to take his place." Sullivan did write,
and Vice President Bush accepted the invitation.

The scene at the Morehouse dedication ceremony when Bush
arrived spoke to the complexity of racial politics at that moment
in time. Across the street from the plaza where Bush was speaking, a crowd of protestors had gathered. But in the overflow audience listening to the vice president were the elite among Atlanta's
Black political figures, all of them Democrats, many of them
prominent civil rights leaders: John Lewis, Andy Young, Julian
Bond, Maynard Jackson, and others. It was, said, Sullivan, "a
highly ecumenical, bi-partisan scene."[6] Afterwards, the Black dig-
nitaries clustered around the vice president for a photo op and a
moment to chat. Bush's entourage kept trying to get him into his
limousine, but he wouldn't go. It was obvious he was enjoying the
event immensely.

Given the Reagan administration's record on social welfare
programs and civil rights enforcement, the scene in front of Morehouse School of Medicine's new building might have seemed in-
congruous to some, even bizarre. But the Black leaders clearly
didn't see it that way. They were proud of the new school and
pleased that, in sending the vice president, the administration
was demonstrating support for more Black physicians and for
improving Black health and health care. As for Vice President
Bush, he and the Bush family had a history in race relations
that most of the Black political figures weren't likely to have
known.

For George H. W. Bush himself that history went back to the
end of World War II when he was mustered out of the Navy after
serving as a combat pilot in the Pacific (and famously being shot

down and rescued). He enrolled as a freshman at Yale shortly afterward, and while he was a student there he had been approached by William Trent, one of the founders of the United Negro College Fund (UNCF). Trent was organizing college support groups for the new Black organization, and Bush volunteered to become UNCF's campus coordinator at Yale. Subsequently Bush and his wife, Barbara, became long-term social friends with Trent and his wife, a highly unusual cross-racial relationship, especially in the elite white circles the Bushes were part of. Few people knew this, and few knew that the Bush family regularly sent sizable, unsolicited donations to UNCF and to Black colleges individually. Their philanthropy wasn't something the Bushes publicized, even when it might have helped Bush politically. "That would be tooting our own horn," Barbara Bush said later. "And we do *not* toot our own horn!"[7]

Not long after his appearance at Morehouse, Vice President Bush invited Sullivan to accompany him, Barbara, and others on an official visit to eight sub-Saharan African nations. In the course of this two-week tour, Sullivan and Barbara Bush developed a warm friendship, and on the way back, Sullivan asked if she would join Morehouse's board of directors. "Something about the mission of the school resonated with me," she said.[8] When the vice president had no objections, she joined Sullivan's board, which gave a prominent name and celebrity firepower to the school's fundraising efforts. When Morehouse embarked on a $15 million national fundraising campaign, Barbara Bush crisscrossed the country with Sullivan, which cemented their friendship and raised the money. Sullivan and his wife, Ginger, found themselves invited to parties and get-togethers at the vice president's residence in Washington, and Bush and Sullivan developed their own relationship.

Six years after Bush's appearance at the Morehouse building dedication, Ronald Reagan's second term was coming to an end, and George Bush gained the Republican presidential nomination. During the planning of the Republican convention, where Bush would be formally nominated, there was a question about who would introduce Barbara Bush, the potential first lady. High-profile names were batted around, but Bush ended up asking Sullivan. "She likes working with you," Bush told Sullivan. "Frankly, I don't even know if you're a Democrat or Republican, but I don't care. Would you do it?"

Sullivan was flattered, and he was pleased to have an opportunity to do something for the board member who had done so much for the medical school. It was Sullivan's first appearance on a political stage. Few of the delegates had any idea who he was.

Three months later Bush was elected president, beating Michael Dukakis. As Bush went about choosing his cabinet, Sullivan found his name mentioned in newspaper speculation about who might be in the running for secretary of Health and Human Services. That took him by surprise; he had no political experience and no political ambition. As far as the public was concerned, he was simply unknown, unlike the leading candidate, C. Everett Koop, who had been President Reagan's high-profile surgeon general for eight years.

When Bush offered him the job, Sullivan thought long and hard before deciding to accept. After thirteen years as dean or president of Morehouse School of Medicine, he still hadn't accomplished everything he had set out to do. The student body was growing, but it was only halfway to what he considered the optimal number. The school covered the major medical specialties but was still working toward incorporating some of the smaller ones, like ophthalmology and dermatology. There were still plenty of hard academic and financial challenges ahead, which he was reluctant to leave in anyone else's hands.

On the other hand, the opportunities presented by the secretaryship were vast. He had been driven all these years since leaving Boston by the goal of creating a greater pool of Black doctors to serve those without decent health care. Morehouse was his avenue toward that goal. AMHPS was a way of building a more powerful means to the same end, and a way to enlarge the concept. Improving African American health didn't just mean more physicians, it meant more dentists, more pharmacists, more veterinarians—the whole range of health professionals. Margaret Heckler in her report had expanded even that concept. Black health wasn't the only issue, she had said, the issue was Black health and *minority* health. And Sullivan, Satcher, and the other AMHPS leaders had embraced that as well.

The HHS secretary position would enable him to pursue the same goals he had been pursuing, but as part of a far more comprehensive portfolio. NIH, CDC, FDA, HRSA (Health Resources and Services Administration), Medicare/Medicaid, and Social Security Administration all came under the Department of Health and Human Services. In one way or another HHS touched every American every day. Here was an opportunity to improve health prospects not just for African Americans or minorities, but for the rest of the nation as well.

Before Bush offered him the job, the two men had rarely, if ever, discussed health policy. But when he visited the White House to talk about the position, Sullivan had laid out some of his basic priorities. There needed to be more diversity among doctors and other health professionals, he told the president-elect. Minorities were grossly underrepresented. More women had to be in senior positions. Minority health problems were a grave concern. Medicaid and other health programs needed to be enlarged.

"I'd support you on those things," Bush had said.

Severing his relationship with Morehouse—federal ethics rule required that—would be hard. Who would replace him? What would their priorities be? Would he feel he had abandoned what he had regarded for years now as a lifetime calling? AMHPS he could leave more comfortably. David Satcher, Walter Bowie, and other leaders there were committed, energetic, highly competent people.

If he took the job, he'd have to be careful not to appear to have any conflicts of interest. Showing bias toward the AMHPS institutions would undercut his credibility, his effectiveness, and whatever moral authority he might have as secretary. On the other hand, AMHPS's objectives were still his objectives. It wasn't clear to him exactly how he might promote those aims even while keeping the association itself at arm's length. But he'd understand that better, he thought, once he got his bearings in Washington.

CHAPTER 8

The Office of Minority Health

The Department of Health and Human Services was vast. With 125,000 employees, its annual budget of $600 billion was the fourth largest in the world, exceeded only by the budgets of the US government, Japan, and the Soviet Union; then, when the Soviet Union collapsed, it became the world's third largest budget. With only his experience at Morehouse School of Medicine as a guide, the immediate question for Sullivan was how to understand and manage such a behemoth. In terms of scale, he was in a different universe.

Sullivan met with the department's senior leaders, and then toured the regional offices, introducing himself to employees around the country and enlisting their support. At the same time, he was thinking hard about his goals and priorities. For the past fourteen years he had devoted his energies to building Morehouse School of Medicine, then AMHPS, and to creating avenues to better the health of the nation's Black community, suffering from its long history of inequitable care. But as head of HHS, a host of other concerns were on his plate, none more dire than the AIDS epidemic, in full swing as he took office. AIDS, smoking, nutrition, obesity, the country's medical research agenda, food safety, children's health, substance abuse, the environment—the HHS portfolio included all these and more. Given the scope of issues, many of them urgent, where and how was he going to pursue his Morehouse and AMHPS objectives while at the same time steering clear of accusations that he might be biased in favor of those historically Black institutions?

The potential appearance of bias concerned him. For their part, Dale Dirks and the AMHPS leaders had no doubts about the depth of his commitment, but at the same time they never anticipated that one of their own would be sitting in the secretary's chair. It had only been six short years since Sullivan, Meharry's David Satcher, Tuskegee's Walter Bowie, and Drew's Alfred Haynes had trooped into Margaret Heckler's office hoping the HHS secretary might give them a serious hearing. While the AMHPS leaders thought Sullivan's new position might give them greater access and leverage, they also understood that he had a far larger agenda now. They waited to see how he was going to handle this and what it would mean for them.

They didn't have to wait long. To administer his oath of office, Sullivan chose Judge Leon Higginbotham. Higginbothan, the Black Third Circuit Appeals Court judge for Eastern Pennsylvania, had a long history as an outspoken civil rights figure. Choosing Higginbotham signaled where Sullivan's priorities lay and the path he intended to pursue. Barbara Bush attended Sullivan's swearing in, along with the president, an unusual thing for her to do. For anyone who might have been looking for signs, the optics told their own story: a civil rights judge, an African American appointee, a presidential couple's friendship.

From the start, Sullivan began remaking the department. He had told President-elect Bush that there needed to be more diversity at HHS and in the health professions generally, that women and minorities were grossly underrepresented. He had said that minority health would be one of his priorities. Bush had said he was in favor. He was "comfortable" with those priorities. The AMHPS leaders may not have been aware of that conversation, but they saw that one of Sullivan's first acts as secretary was to appoint a group to look at all of the department's scientific and public health advisory committees to see how integrated they were and make recommendations for recruitment.

To head the committee, Sullivan appointed Bill Bennett, the African American Bureau of Manpower official who had been so helpful to Morehouse College president Hugh Gloster when he started planning the medical school. From Bennett's committee Sullivan got a bank of potential candidates, a diverse group who were ready to fill slots as they opened up.

Sullivan also looked at senior positions. In its upper echelons, HHS was practically all male and lily-white, as it always had been. But that didn't last. Sullivan brought in Bernadine Healy, a renowned cardiologist and researcher at the Cleveland Clinic, to serve as NIH's first female director. He tapped Gwendolyn King for social security commissioner, also the first woman. Healy was white; King, Black.

He brought in Bill Toby to head the Health Care Financing Administration. Toby, also African American, was a long-term official in HHS's Region 2 New York office. Ronny Lancaster, an African American attorney, came to Washington as principal deputy assistant secretary for planning and evaluation.

To replace Koop as surgeon general, Sullivan turned to Antonia Novello, a Puerto Rican physician who was serving as deputy director of the NIH Institute of Child Health and Human Development. Novello was the first woman and first minority person to be named surgeon general, the nation's top doctor. Sullivan presented these names to Bush, who formally nominated those who needed Senate confirmation. There was no opposition in Congress. Nor, as the department's complexion began to shift, were there any hints of pushback or resentment at HHS.

To most observers, the changes Sullivan was implementing seemed appropriate. Diversity had entered the national discussion with President Lyndon Johnson's Great Society programs and emerged as a headline issue in 1978 when the Supreme Court decided in the Bakke case (*Regents of the University of California v. Bakke*) that diversity was beneficial to medical schools, and by implication, to other institutions as well. But Sullivan's personnel moves had more than a general cultural effect. They were strategic.

Bernadine Healy wasn't just the first female director, she was an activist, a prominent voice on issues of women in medicine and health care for women. Along with other women medical scientists she was unhappy that women's opinions tended to be disregarded by their male colleagues, and she was anything but reticent. She brought attention to the paucity of women enrollees in clinical trials. Trials on medicines and other therapies typically enrolled men (typically white men), the assumption being that the results would apply to women as well. Heart disease in women, for example, was not well-studied (Healy was a cardiologist), one result being that women transported to hospitals with heart attacks were often misdiagnosed. Their symptoms were frequently different from men's symptoms, confusing male doctors who tended to ascribe women's complaints to emotional causes, which delayed or precluded therapeutic measures. Having more women at the table when research decisions were being made would help address the badly neglected needs of women's health. Healy was a leader in that cause.

By the same token, appointing African Americans to senior management roles and scientific advisory positions would advance the agenda of minority health. Black health issues were now going to be given greater attention and support. The HHS agencies were put on notice that the secretary was serious about resolving health status disparities and increasing the number of minority physicians and other health professionals.

Sullivan was aware he was taking a chance that his primary mission might be seen as racially oriented, not an impression he wanted to convey. But the reality was that the people who were most impacted by poor health and inadequate care were poor people, white as well as Black, and far more whites than Blacks, though the poverty *rate* was higher in the Black community. Other priorities loomed large—AIDS most urgently. The Reagan administration had done its best to avoid engaging with sex-related issues. Sullivan, with Bush's support, planned a multipronged, multibillion-dollar effort to counter the disease. But Sullivan's engagement with the poor and minorities was unmistakable. That was the direction he was going; it was the tenor of his agenda.

~

To the extent that the AMHPS leadership harbored any lingering doubts about their relationship with the new HHS secretary, their doubts were alleviated when soon after his appointment, Sullivan was asked to give the keynote address at a National Health Council meeting. At the meeting were two hundred people from major health-related organizations (such as the American Cancer Society, the American Heart Association, the American Diabetes Association, and the American Lung Association), physician associations, the insurance and pharmaceutical industries, research agencies, policy think tanks, and congressional staffs. Sullivan had arranged for Dale Dirks to sit at the head table with him. He recognized Dirks specifically and spoke briefly about the importance of AMHPS. To anyone looking on, the message was loud and clear.

AMHPS had had decent access to the national health organizations as well as to NIH before Sullivan's appointment. The association's close relationship with Louis Stokes was common knowledge, as was its working relationship with other powerful congressional figures. In addition, the Heckler Report of 1985 was still relatively fresh in people's minds, and the agencies were looking to respond positively if they could.

But with Sullivan heading HHS, AMHPS's access to government health institutions increased considerably. The changed atmosphere encouraged the agencies, and they started to find ways to work with the AMHPS institutions that would not have occurred to them earlier. The new secretary was making it clear that the AMHPS schools were a resource for ideas and advice, and that eased their access.

Dirks recalled:

> You'd walk into an agency, and you'd be greeted with open arms. . . .
> Our members might be sitting around a table in our conference
> room talking about what agencies we were working to persuade on
> one issue or another and which ones we needed to see, the Centers
> for Disease Control, for example. We'd get in touch with the CDC
> director's office, and a few days later we'd be sitting down with the
> individuals we wanted to talk to. We'd take our deans and presi-
> dents, and we'd walk out of there with ten different ideas on how
> the agency could work with our institutions to conduct program
> activity. Only a few years back that would have been a pipe dream.[1]

Sullivan encouraged the AMHPS schools to send resumes of faculty members and leaders to the NIH institutes so their people could be selected to serve on advisory councils and study sections. NIH relied on its peer review system to make decisions about which research proposals to fund and which to decline. But if a grant proposal went to a study section that included no actual peers of the researcher submitting the proposal, the concept to be studied might well seem difficult to understand, or worse, unimportant. But if a study section included someone with a background in studying minority health, that proposal, perhaps from a Meharry or Tuskegee or Xavier researcher, might well find more traction. And this began to happen.

In all of this, Sullivan was careful to follow ethical guidelines. But the fact was that he never had to intervene personally. His position as secretary exerted its own inevitable force. Beyond that, it was well known that there was a warm relationship between him and President and Mrs. Bush, which provided its own aura. The structural changes Sullivan initiated encouraged NIH, CDC, and the other health agencies under HHS to view Black and minority health issues with greater responsiveness. In the new HHS environment, studies on disparities in care, the paucity of minority health professionals, and the nature of Black morbidity and mortality gained significance and legitimacy.

In addition, Sullivan's former partners at the AMHPS institutions maintained their contacts with him even though there was now no formal relationship. David Satcher, Walter Bowie, Tony Rachal, and others spoke with him often, giving him their perspective on what was going on among their colleagues and in the field. They gave him feedback on how programs were performing, what areas needed greater emphasis or more support, what controversies were emerging, and how he, or the department, might help to resolve them.

~

The years prior to Sullivan's appointment had been productive for AMHPS in unforeseen ways. In particular, the institutions had found support for their objectives on both sides of the aisle, from conservatives as well as from liberals. The legislation AMHPS had initiated and helped draft, often in partnership with Louis Stokes's office, had struck a responsive chord among a broad ideological range of legislators, this even as Democrats and Republicans were engaged in hard conflicts on other issues. Unprecedented legislation that funneled money to Black institutions in order to improve health care for African Americans had passed with very little opposition, sometimes on simple voice votes. Those successes were partly due to the strategic acumen of AMHPS's leaders and partly to the association's relentless lobbying. But all that had fallen on fertile congressional ground.

The years 1986 through 1988 had been richly productive. And now Sullivan was in the secretary's chair, operating there with apparently solid presidential backing. Congressman Stokes took stock of this situation—the bipartisanship, the new regime at HHS, the president's support—and decided the time was right to raise the effort to the next level. Stokes was chair of the Congressional Black Caucus's Health Brain Trust; he was the second-ranking Democrat on the House Appropriations Committee. He had known and worked with Sullivan since 1975 when Atlanta representative Andy Young brought the then newly minted medical school dean to meet him—fourteen years before. Since then the two Louises had developed a warm, personal relationship, as well as an effortless working partnership. To Stokes, all this meant the momentum was there to build on what he and AMHPS had already accomplished. The stars for it were in alignment. He looked at the Black Graduate Institutions program, the Excellence in Minority Health Education and Care Act, the Research Centers in Minority Institutions program, and he thought: now is the time to up the ante.

AMHPS had been hammering away on the policy front regarding training more minorities in the health professions to bring essential care to underserved areas, which would improve the grim state of minority health and benefit mainstream health at the same time. That message, repeated in forum after forum and in congressional office after congressional office, seemed to have taken hold, at least among members of Congress who were significantly concerned about health policy.

The three major pieces of legislation already in place had strengthened the AMHPS schools in a variety of ways. The most pressing next step, Stokes and the AMHPS leaders decided, was to find a mechanism to assist minority students who wanted to pursue careers in the health professions but were prevented by the costs involved. That was the primary thrust of the Disadvantaged Minority Health Improvement Act, introduced in 1989. David Satcher, Walter Bowie, and Marcellus Grace worked with Stokes and Dirks to craft the legislation. Bowie had served as AMHPS president after Sullivan, and now Grace was filling that role. Stokes and Henry Waxman sponsored the bill in the House; Ted Kennedy introduced the Senate version.

The AMHPS schools had received support that improved their financial viability and their status as centers for learning and research. Now Congress authorized tuition scholarships for students from disadvantaged backgrounds. To facilitate the utilization of these funds, grants were made directly to the schools, which then were able to offer scholarships to students. Talented undergraduates from low-income homes who had likely already accumulated loan debt to attend college, and who might have felt compelled to enter the workforce, now had the ability to go on to medical or dental, pharmacy or veterinary school instead. The act gave the health profession schools a deeper pool of prospective students. For the schools and for many undergraduates, it was a game changer.

The act also reauthorized a program that reached down into undergraduate and secondary schools to identify and prepare minority students who showed academic talent and were potential candidates for careers in health. It provided funds for information and counseling, for mentors and summer or part-time clinical experience. Sullivan had told President-elect Bush that minorities were grossly underrepresented in the health professions. That was partly due to the straightened circumstances of the Black training institutions and partly due to the traditional exclusions and biases of the mainstream schools. But it was also due to the inadequate preparation and awareness of many African American students as they proceeded through high school and college. The act's Health Careers Opportunity Program didn't nearly resolve that problem, but it took important steps in the right direction.

The Disadvantaged Minority Health Improvement Act enlarged the pipeline for prospective health professionals; it helped students identify career choices, and it provided money to help them realize their aspirations. At the same time the act looked at the faculty side of the equation. The AMHPS schools were not just constrained in terms of the pool of prospective students, they were also constrained when it came to hiring faculty. In this area their resources often didn't permit them to successfully compete for talent. Many minority individuals in the academic arena would have loved to teach at a Meharry or a Morehouse and make a contribution to the mission of improving Black health. But the predominantly Black institutions frequently did not have the financial resources to offer the kind of salaries that the larger academic health centers could.

The act addressed this issue by creating a minority faculty educational-loan repayment program that enabled a Meharry or Tuskegee or Xavier to offer prospective faculty hires forgiveness of their educational loans. For promising young academics from disadvantaged backgrounds, this was a significant monetary incentive that often allowed them to accept jobs at Black institutions that otherwise they couldn't afford to.

The Disadvantaged Minority Health Improvement Act created these new monetary programs that advanced the ability of minority schools to attract students and faculty. At the same time, the act reauthorized the Centers of Excellence in Minority Health program. "It wasn't as all-encompassing as I would have liked," Stokes said later, "but it was substantial . . . the first comprehensive legislation addressing minority health ever passed by the US Congress. It was a landmark."[2] The bill passed both the House and Senate by voice vote. There were no dissenters. Sullivan recommended it to President Bush, who signed it on October 10, 1990. The entire process, from drafting to enactment, had taken less than a year.

To those involved, the new act may have seemed simply an extension of the previous string of legislative accomplishments, the logical next step in an ongoing dynamic of government support for minority health professions schools. But from a historical perspective, it's easier to see the groundbreaking nature of the AMHPS-driven legislation of those years. For centuries the health of Black people in America had been regarded as inconsequential, or worse. Against a past when ingrained customs and racist convictions had placed roadblocks to the progress of Blacks in medicine and to Black health care, the minority health professions legislation of 1986 through 1990 marked a historic about face. For the first time since Reconstruction, the US government was acknowledging, in some degree at least, its responsibility for the health of the country's minority citizens. It was not looking at the root causes of the terrible health disparities between Black and white Americans, and it was not yet facing up to the grave deficiencies of health insurance coverage. But it *was* providing meaningful support for the thin line of Black health professions schools upon which so much depended. (In 2021 these programs still exist and are still meaningful.)

When Sullivan came into office and began educating himself about the history of NIH, he saw that its institutes and centers had come into being in a variety of ways, and several had been established only shortly before his appointment. One, the National Institute on Deafness, had been created in 1988, only a year before he became secretary; the National Center for Nursing Research just two years before that. The Institute on Deafness had been precipitated by Senator Tom Harkin, whose brother was deaf. The nursing center was also a political creation, proposed and championed by Illinois representative Edward Madigan. These and various other NIH offices, centers, and institutes had been established because a well-placed individual was particularly interested and pressed for the creation of a focused research entity. That is, they were initiated *politically* rather than, for example, as the result of a *scientific* decision based on medical research priorities.

The issue of how disease affects minorities was high on Sullivan's agenda. African Americans had high incidences of heart disease, diabetes, cancer, and hypertension relative to white Americans. Why was that? NIH research on minority health was minimal. In terms of funding, it was barely an afterthought. Did these issues, he thought, not warrant their own place as an NIH entity?

When he understood he had the power to establish an office for minority health to further investigate these and other racially-based health issues, Sullivan worked with Ruth Kirschstein (NIH's acting director before Bernadine Healy's appointment), who agreed with him about the need. At his urging, Kirschstein established an office of minority programs within the NIH director's office. Kirschstein then initiated a search for a director of the new entity.

~

It didn't take long before Kirschstein and Sullivan settled on John Ruffin. Ruffin was a biologist. He had a PhD from Kansas State

University and had done postdoctoral work at Harvard. Ruffin was chair of the biology department and dean of the School of Arts and Sciences at North Carolina Central University. He knew the historically Black colleges and universities well; he had taught at several of them. He also knew NIH, having served on various NIH review committees and work groups. "When you come to work for NIH," Sullivan told him, "it's my expectation that you will have a seat at the table equal to any other associate director." (That turned out to be more than a little optimistic.) Kirschstein and Sullivan were impressed by Ruffin's academic and administrative qualifications. He also seemed resilient and determined, qualities that were going to be severely tested in his new office.

When Ruffin started his job, Sullivan briefed him about what he expected. The mission, Sullivan said, was twofold. First, was to focus on disparities, in terms of disease, in terms of care, in terms of longevity. Why did Blacks suffer from those disparities? What could be done about it? Second, there were far too few Black physicians and medical scientists. If there were more doctors and dentists, there would be better care. If there were more investigators, there would be more attention and greater understanding. How could prospective minority health professionals be better identified, recruited, and trained? Sullivan wanted Ruffin to take that double charge and run with it.

The years since Heckler's report had seen the country waking up to the issue of disparate minority health. At bottom, unequal care meant very simply that Black lives were valued less than white lives. African Americans suffered more from disease; they died at greater rates; they lived shorter lives. The same attention was not given to their lives as it was to white lives. The US government had acknowledged this as a national concern with the Heckler Report; it had taken certain steps to address the problem with legislation. Now, with the newly established Office for Minority Health and with John Ruffin's appointment, the government had brought on a point person to push for—even to galvanize, Sullivan hoped—a response at the country's premier institute for health science investigation.

Back in 1983, Sullivan, Satcher, Bowie, and Haynes had left the AMHPS white paper—*Blacks and the Health Professions in the '80s: A National Crisis and a Time for Action*—on Margaret Heckler's desk. That report had focused on two critical issues: unequal care and the dire shortage of Black health professionals. Now, seven years later, Sullivan was handing exactly those issues to a formally appointed program director at NIH and telling him the time had come to bring the country's medical science resources to bear.

That was progress, albeit very slow progress. It brought on line a full-time, high-level official whose job it was to address minority health care and professional training. At the very same time, though, that official's field of action was cramped and constricted. Sullivan had the authority to create an office but not to fund it or accord it broad powers. The terms of Ruffin's office stipulated that he had no ability to make grants himself. If he wanted to further research, he needed to find a partner in one of NIH's established institutes to do it for him, which made his effectiveness dependent on the goodwill of others. Not only did Ruffin have no grantmaking authority, he had no money to distribute or to exercise leverage in other ways. His budget when he stepped into office was $1.5 million—in NIH terms, hardly enough to warrant the term "pittance." Ruffin was in office; but with no budget and no authority, he was essentially powerless. "I asked myself," Ruffin remembers, "what can I do with one and a half million dollars?"[3]

His answer was to create a fact-finding committee to reach out to communities of color and to the biomedical establishment in order to define underlying causes of disparities and to elicit solutions to the paucity of minorities in the health professions. Ruffin appointed as cochairs of this fact-finding group David Satcher, president of Meharry, and Norman Francis, president of Xavier University. Both men were founders of AMHPS and pillars in the association's efforts. They had spent a great deal of energy over many years in building AMHPS. Moreover, Satcher was AMHPS's current president. There was little difference between his priorities as president and those he and Francis were helping Ruffin define.

At the conclusion of its work, the Satcher/Francis group gave Ruffin a report that listed thirteen recommendations. Nine of the thirteen had to do with expanding the number of minority students in the biomedical sciences—the AMHPS schools' priority from the association's beginning. AMHPS recommendations were thus built into the goals of Ruffin's office.

~

Ruffin had built his career as a bench scientist and teacher, then as an administrator. Although he was not a trained historian, he understood that he was in the middle of something historic. Ruffin was now, in fact, at the heart of the federal government's commitment to improve minority health and eliminate disparities. In this work he had powerful allies—Satcher, Stokes, Sullivan, and others. But his office was in the eye of the storm. Ruffin's allies, those he could unreservedly count on, were few. Inside NIH, there was acting director Ruth Kirschstein, and then Bernadine Healy when she took over as director. Meanwhile, those who needed persuading were many. Many, or most, of the Institute directors, whose buy-in Ruffin needed if he were to advance his agenda—were not convinced that minority health should be a priority for their institutes.

As a result, Ruffin embarked on his long journey as director (he served from 1990 until his retirement in 2015) in something of a schizophrenic atmosphere: enthusiasm and support on one side countered by stubbornness and skepticism on the other.

The support emanated from Sullivan's leadership at HHS and Healy's at NIH. With Sullivan as secretary, the Department of Health and Human Services had reoriented itself with regard to minority issues. AMHPS was now more a force than it had ever been. At NIH Healy was a passionate advocate, not just for women's health issues but also for minority health. Additionally, in 1991 Louis Stokes became what was known as a "cardinal," chair of an appropriations subcommittee, which made him one of the most powerful members of Congress.

In this atmosphere Congress appropriated $45 million for the development of research initiatives on various dimensions of minority health and for programs to increase the number of minority researchers in the biomedical sciences. This level of funding was little more than a rounding error in NIH terms. And because Ruffin had no grantmaking authority himself, he had to work with the various institutes in terms of distributing the money. But funding was funding, and this money helped lay a foundation at NIH for minority health programs.

Ruffin was an effective advocate in his own cause, and some of the NIH's institutes and centers responded positively to his proposals and suggestions. He later wrote that the $45 million that funded his Minority Health Initiative "was the one achievement . . . that encountered the least resistance at NIH, because it had support at the highest level."[4] Ruffin was also sometimes effective at creating a positive environment for grant proposals coming to the Institutes from minority investigators. He was able to go to his colleagues at the various institutes and centers and say, this area or that looks like it would make real advances if a few more grant proposals were funded. To which the director of that institute or center might say, "You know, I'm not sure that's important." Or, less likely, "Yes, that makes a lot of sense."

In these things Ruffin frequently worked closely with AMHPS. In most important areas, their agendas were identical. AMHPS brought leverage from the outside; Ruffin's office was within the NIH director's office, which gave him a degree of prominence inside the Institutes. "We'd meet with Ruffin," Dirks recalled, "to ask him to press a particular institute for some program. We'd say, 'How can we help advance your initiatives on this or that?' And, 'By the way, here are the resumes of fifteen faculty members that we've gathered. Can you talk with your NIH colleagues and ask them to consider including these people on advisory councils or study sections?'"[5]

Ruffin was a collegial and persuasive man, but having an administratively established position within the director's office was a double-edged sword. The NIH director (acting director Kirschstein at the time) had created the office by fiat. Healy was every bit as supportive as her predecessor, but another director might decide an office on minority health wasn't needed and could abolish it with the stroke of a pen. Now and then the NIH directorship changed hands, so that was a danger. National elections were also a danger. In 1992 Bill Clinton defeated George H. W. Bush, which meant that Louis Sullivan's tenure as HHS secretary was over. Clinton brought in as secretary Donna Shalala, who was a friend to Ruffin and his office. But Shalala's NIH director, Harold Varmus, was no ally at all.

To preclude any problems that might develop regarding the preservation of Ruffin's office, in 1993 Stokes and Ted Kennedy sponsored the NIH Health Revitalization Act that established both the office of women's health and the office of minority health on a statutory basis. In addition, the act created the opportunity for AMHPS institutions accessing the funding set aside by the 1987

Excellence in Minority Health Education and Care Act to be designated as "Institutions of Emerging Excellence," thus providing
opportunities for these institutions to access NIH-supported extramural research facilities grants. AMHPS was heavily involved
in the drafting, along with Kennedy and Stokes.

Ruffin's office was now permanent. Neither Varmus nor any
future NIH director would be able to threaten its existence. But
Ruffin was still hamstrung, with a minimal budget and no grant-
making authority, which meant he was as dependent on the directors of NIH's twenty-three institutes, as he had always been. And
here he was facing headwinds.

～

The first problem was that the Office of Research on Minority
Health was an orphan. The NIH's twenty-three institutes were in
a sense a family whose parent was the NIH director. Some of these
institutes had been created through outside political pressure, as
Sullivan had seen when he originally established Ruffin's office.
But most were outgrowths of needs expressed by NIH internally—
the National Human Genome Research Institute, for example.
NIH had wanted a research entity to map out the human genome.
NIH and the National Academy of Sciences asked Congress for
authorization and funding. Congress responded by establishing
an office. Further requests for support raised the "office" to a "center," and finally to an "institute"—NIH's most prestigious and
best-funded level.

The Office of Research on Minority Health was not a legitimate
NIH family member in the sense that the Genome Research Institute was. Ruffin's office was formalized by legislative action
because both the House and Senate had recognized that America's minorities were subject to disease and death to a far greater
degree than mainstream Americans. Congress voted to establish
an office in order to address that. NIH was not asking Congress

to do this; Congress was telling NIH to do it. In other words, Ruffin's office (and mandate) was imposed from the outside. At various
levels throughout the NIH, this did not sit well. During Sullivan's
tenure, negative feelings on this subject were suppressed. But many
in NIH leadership positions saw little need for a minority health
office. Some, immersed in their own research, seemed to Ruffin
"largely oblivious to the existence of the disparities my office had
been established to address."[6]

~

But Ruffin's problems went beyond the sense that his office was
outside the family. The whole idea of research on minority health
clashed with NIH's deep culture.

Most of the NIH institutes and centers were focused on specific
diseases or conditions: the Cancer Institute on cancer; the Heart,
Lung, and Blood Institute on diseases of those organs; the Institute of Neurological Disorders and Stroke on problems in those
areas. Others had to do with specific fields: research on drug abuse,
child development, alcoholism, aging, etc. In each of these fields,
the general direction of research was guided by "scientific advisory councils," while specific grant proposals were evaluated by
study sections.

Within this framework, grant proposals were judged by rele-
vance to the particular institute's priorities and by the elegance
and substantive potential of the proposal. But the institutes were
all focused on research in their own fields. For no institute was disparities in health care a prominent concern, or (for most) any
concern at all. A proposal regarding heart disease statistics among
Black women as compared with white women might have little
chance for success at the Heart, Lung, and Blood Institute. A study
limited to heart disease among Black women might have a better
chance of being reviewed, but probably would not do well against
similar proposals aimed at women in general, whose results would

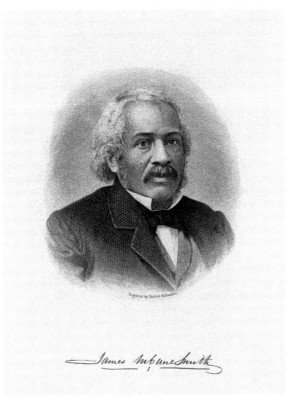

James McCune Smith. "We are in for the fight and will fight it out here." Patrick H. Reason, *James McCune Smith*, engraving, ca. 1850.

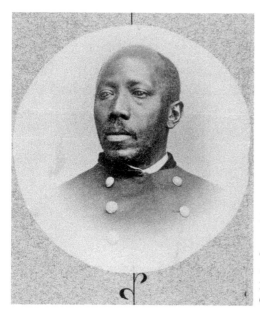

Martin Robison Delany.
"I weary of our miserable
condition."
(Courtesy of US Army
Heritage and Education
Center)

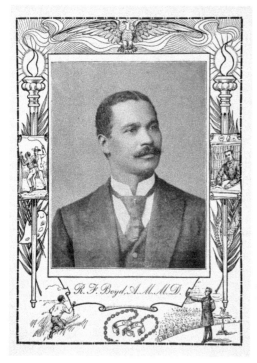

Robert Fulton Boyd.
First president of the
National Medical
Association. "R. F. Boyd,
A. M. M. D."
(The New York Public Library
Digital Collections, 1902,
https://digitalcollections.
nypl.org/items/510d
47da-75fa-a3d9-e040
-e00a18064a99.)

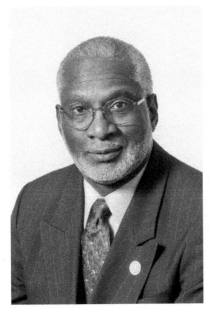

Dr. David Satcher. Surgeon General; Assistant Secretary, Department of Health and Human Services; Director, Centers for Disease Control and Prevention; founding board member of AMHPS.
(Courtesy of David Satcher)

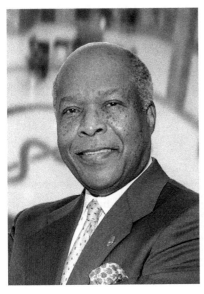

Dr. Louis W. Sullivan. Founding Dean and President, Morehouse School of Medicine; Secretary, Department of Health and Human Services; founding board member of AMHPS.
(Courtesy of Louis Sullivan)

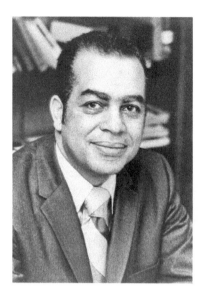

Dr. Lloyd Elam. President, Meharry Medical College; founding board member of AMHPS. (Courtesy of Meharry Medical College)

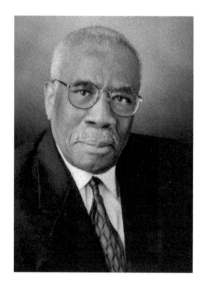

Dr. Walter Bowie. Dean, Tuskegee School of Veterinary Medicine; founding board member of AMHPS. (Courtesy of Tuskegee College of Veterinary Medicine)

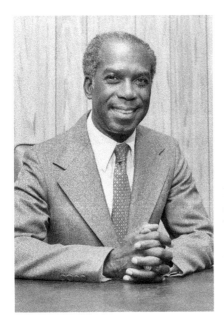

Dr. Alfred Haynes. President, Charles R. Drew University of Medicine and Science; founding board member of AMHPS.
(Courtesy of Charles R. Drew University of Medicine and Science)

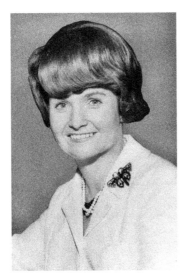

Margaret Heckler. Secretary, Department of Health and Human Services. In 1985 she released the *Report of the Secretary's Task Force on Black and Minority Health.*
(Collection US House of Representatives)

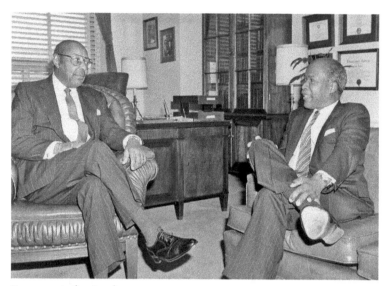

Representative Louis
Stokes (*left*) and Health and
Human Services Secretary
Dr. Louis Sullivan (*right*).
(Courtesy of Louis Stokes)

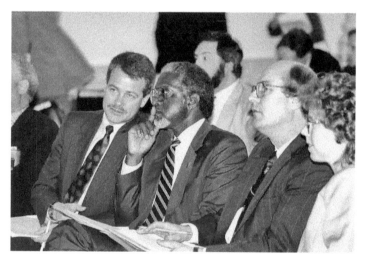

Dale Dirks (*far left*) and
Dr. David Satcher conferring
during a congressional hearing.
(AMHPS Collection)

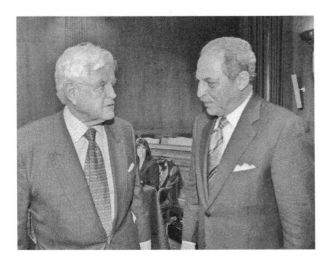

Senator Ted Kennedy and
Meharry Medical College
president and president
of AMHPS John Maupin.
(Courtesy of John Maupin)

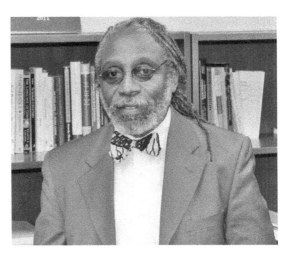

Dr. Rueben Warren.
Dean, Meharry Medi-
cal College School of
Dentistry; Director,
Tuskegee University
National Center for
Bioethics in Research
and Health Care;
Associate Director,
CDC; board member
of AMHPS.
(Courtesy of Rueben
Warren)

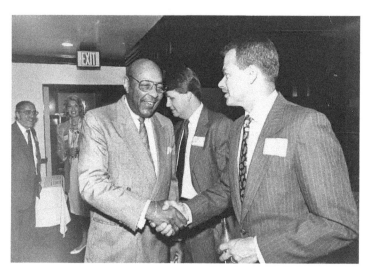

Louis Stokes and Dale Dirks.
(AMHPS Collection)

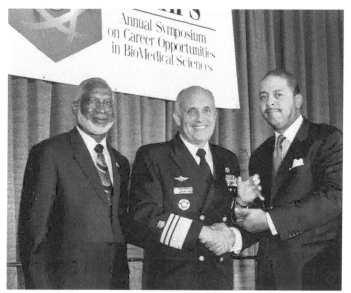

From left: Dr. David Satcher; Surgeon General Richard Carmona; and Ronny Lancaster, president of AMHPS.
(AMHPS Collection)

have broader applicability. Health disparities were not a priority at the institute, nor were diseases specific to Black women.

It was here that John Ruffin's powers of persuasion were tested. He needed to stay as collegial as possible, yet at the same time make his strongest case for studies that furthered his office's priorities. This was a challenge he faced nearly every day. Dirks watched this tightrope dance for the entire first decade of Ruffin's tenure—from 1990 to 2000, when the Office of Research on Minority Health was upgraded to a center, which gave Ruffin his own budget. Reflecting on the period following Healy's brief stint as director, Dirks commented, "Ruffin probably never had a meeting with the director of NIH where the director said something like, 'I like the direction you're taking.' He never had one of those meetings. It was always more like, 'Gosh, John, you know how it is. The institutes are all going in one direction, and here you want to go in another.' Ruffin fought that battle every single day."[7]

It was also a fact that when it came to judging grant requests, proposals from researchers at AMHPS institutions were at a disadvantage from the start. Sometimes their proposals were for studies outside the primary concerns of the NIH institute or center considering them. When they were judged to be focused and relevant, they entered a highly selective peer review process. Peer review was the NIH gold standard, never deviated from, and considered the single valid approach for allocating limited resources to the best quality proposals. But the best quality proposals tended to come from the most prominent investigators at the most highly regarded institutions, from the Harvards and Stanfords and Columbias, not from the Meharrys and Xaviers and Tuskegees with their sparse records of scientific research.

But Ruffin understood that he had been appointed to serve a constituency, and his constituency was the minority population and the minority health institutions that served them. With that agenda he knew he could not be confined by the usual way NIH did business. The topic of disparities in health care did not have a natural home at NIH. The peer review system favored the usual suspects. Ruffin's job, as he saw it, was to raise the level of the minority institutions, to nurture their medical scientists, to help them become more experienced and sophisticated, to carve out funding space for their concerns, and to awaken the science-minded NIH world to the realities of disparate care. That, and to give the Black community the wherewithal to care for its own, denied them by their history of conflict with the racial antipathies that had always impeded and blocked their efforts. There was, then, continual tension between what Ruffin wanted and what the conservative inertia of the institutes imposed.

Beyond that was the subtle question of racism, never obvious, but always hovering off on the periphery. Ruffin would argue that a grant proposal to study Blacks and diabetes was important, and the answer would come, "We're working on diabetes studies that are as relevant to Blacks as to whites. We don't think we need a separate study on Blacks." And so that subtle hint of racism would suddenly seem more noticeable.

But here Ruffin had to tread with extraordinary care. He needed buy-in not pushback, and so he kept his peace. It was only years later, after his retirement, that he could say, "Yes, there was an element of that."[8]

~

In spite of all the crosscurrents and shoals he needed to navigate, Ruffin was successful at putting minorities on the advisory committees and study sections. His working relationships with many of the NIH institutes did produce results. As relentless as he was, he opened minds to the need to examine disparities in health care and their destructive consequences. Despite his relatively powerless position, his lack of a meaningful budget, and his dependence on others, in his first four years Ruffin emerged as an effective advocate, with help from Stokes and Stokes's congressional allies and from the parallel efforts of AMHPS and the association's senior statesmen—Sullivan, Satcher, Francis, Bowie, Rachal, and others.

But in 1994 the ground under the American political world shook. For more than forty years, the Democrats had controlled the House of Representatives, with its power of the purse—from Dwight Eisenhower to the election of Bill Clinton. Democratic control of the House had come to seem almost a permanent fixture of America's political landscape. But the 1994 midterm election administered a shock to the system. Suddenly the Democrats were out, and Newt Gingrich, with his Contract with America, was in. For almost a decade AMHPS's legislative efforts had thrived on a bipartisan spirit in both House and Senate. With Gingrich as speaker, the political skies darkened.

CHAPTER 9

The Center for Minority Health and Health Disparities

When Louis Sullivan was sworn in as HHS secretary in 1989, he and Newt Gingrich had known each other for many years. Gingrich was elected from Georgia's sixth congressional district in 1978, only three years after Sullivan arrived in Atlanta as Morehouse School of Medicine's founding dean. Gingrich came in from the academic world as a reformer (he was a history professor at West Georgia College), bursting with ideas, championing the principle of equal opportunity—the first Republican to ever hold the seat.

Georgia's sixth included parts of North Atlanta, near Morehouse, and Gingrich and the dean soon got to know each other. Impressed by the new Black medical school and its rapid progress, Gingrich became an enthusiastic supporter, and the two men developed a congenial personal relationship. Their friendship was still in place eleven years later when Sullivan came to Washington to head the Department of Health and Human Services. Shortly after Sullivan arrived, Gingrich came to see him at his new office in the Hubert H. Humphrey Building, offering his help and talking about ways they might work together.

Gingrich was then House minority whip, articulate, combative, known for his scathing denunciation of Democrats. In late day House sessions, often with no other members in their seats, Gingrich held forth on C-SPAN declaring a war of civilizations between virtuous Republicans and treasonous Democrats. Democrats were corrupt, incompetent, pathetic, hypocritical, shallow traitors, descriptive terms he developed into a vocabulary list for Republicans to use in future campaigns.

Gingrich's appetite for political trench warfare wasn't on the new HHS secretary's radar screen. With the exception of minority health issues, prior to his nomination Sullivan had had essentially zero interest in Washington politics. He had come to town as a true outsider, with little feel for the harsh realities of the capital's political life. He did know that Gingrich wasn't on any of the committees directly involved in HHS affairs. So while Sullivan didn't think they'd necessarily have much legislative interaction, he appreciated the offer of support from an old ally who had early on demonstrated his backing for Black medical education and minority affairs in general. Neither man imagined that Gingrich and his group of Republican firebrands would within a few years pose a critical threat to the financial well-being of Morehouse, Meharry, Tuskegee, Xavier, and the other AMHPS schools.

The threat was embodied in Gingrich's Contract with America (President Bill Clinton called it a Contract *on* America), which propelled the Republicans to an avalanche of victories in the 1994 midterm elections. The Senate and the House, both controlled by Democrats, now suddenly flipped and turned Republican. The Republican Senate victory was a surprise but not unprecedented; the upper chamber had changed hands several times in the previous ten years. But the Republican triumph in the House was a political earthquake. There, the Republicans gained fifty-four seats, destroying the Democratic stranglehold that had been in place for four decades.

In the Senate, a more collegial place to begin with, the new majority signaled a different direction. But senators knew that one term's majority might be the next term's minority. The fellow committee member who might need to defer to you now could well hold the reins after the next electoral cycle, which exerted a certain restraint on antagonisms. But in the House, the new majority elected Gingrich speaker, and with his rise, scorched-earth ideological warfare descended on the chamber.

The Contract with America listed ten major policy changes that Republicans promised to bring to the House floor. Many of the bills they submitted included elements attractive to Democrats as well as Republicans, but the underlying thrust of the Contract was to radically reduce government spending on everything other than defense. From the point of view of the AMHPS institutions, that augured bad times, and the new Republican House lost no time in fulfilling the AMHPS leaders' fears. The minority health care statutes already in place weren't in danger, but funding for them needed to be approved each year, and that was meat for the Republican fiscal grinder.

If any illustration was needed of Republican intentions, Bob Livingston, the new head of the House Appropriations Committee, brought to his first meeting a Bowie knife, a machete, and an alligator skinning knife (he was from Louisiana), colorful visuals of what he planned to do to the budget. The Labor and Health and Human Services appropriations subcommittee, headed now by Republican John Edward Porter from Illinois, lost no time in filling out the picture.

The "Labor H" subcommittee controlled almost all health-related funding. In the committee's markup of the new spending bill, not only was new funding slashed, but the previous year's appropriations—approved by the then Democratic controlled committee—were laid on the chopping block. *We're not only going to cut spending,* the committee declared as it got down to work; *we're going to go back to the previous fiscal year and roll back those programs too.* The proposed cuts applied to virtually every social program in the Labor H bill; the AMHPS schools weren't the only ones holding their breath. But for them a reduction in funding already approved would be near catastrophic.

The retroactive budget cutting effort proceeded through the House, but the Senate didn't assent; so the previous year's money, at least, was safe. Current and future prospects, though, looked grim.

The funding horizon was bleak. But worse was the toxic atmosphere that spread over the House committees, with its baneful, far-flung consequences, reaching at this writing, well into the twenty-first century. "Amity between Democrats and Republicans was hardly universal before Gingrich," Louis Stokes recalled, "but it wasn't uncommon either. . . . Gingrich put an end to that. His tenure triggered the long pernicious slide into the ferocious partisanship that has gone so far toward ruining decent, effective government."[1]

Stokes, who had championed so much of the minority health care legislation, had his own bitter experience of this. The chief reason he had always been so effective was his ability to reach across the aisle. On his own appropriations subcommittee he had worked closely with his Republican ranking member, Jerry Lewis from California. Although Stokes's and Lewis's positions were often opposed, Stokes's practice had been to consult with Lewis whenever a bill was submitted in order to reduce whatever differences they could. As a result, when it was time to mark up the bill, many conflicts had already been ironed out.

Over time Stokes and Lewis developed a warm personal friendship, as well as an effective working relationship. But when Gingrich took over as speaker, it all came to a sudden halt. With Lewis now chair and Stokes the ranking member, consultation ended. Lewis stopped talking to Stokes about issues, even informally, simply imposing himself instead. In earlier congresses it had been customary for Democratic House committee chairs to take their ranking members with them to conference meetings with Senate counterparts to reconcile differences in House and Senate bills. Now, that ceased as well. "It became rancorous," Stokes said. "I didn't understand it. . . . [W]e had worked closely together for a long time. . . . What in the world had happened to him?"[2]

What had happened was that Gingrich had imposed a loyalty oath on Republican House members. They were sworn to support the Contract, which shut the door on compromise or even consultation. In addition, he banned personal contact between Republicans and Democratic members of Congress, an unprecedented effort to control friendly interactions that might seduce Republicans away from their sworn loyalty.

In Stokes's case, after a period of time, Lewis arranged to have lunch with him, explaining what had happened and apologizing for the change in their relationship. It was likely, he told Stokes, that he was violating Gingrich's ban just in having a meal together. But of course it wasn't just Lewis and Stokes. They weren't the only ones who had worked in a consultative way or had enjoyed some level of friendship. Instead a chill descended on relationships that had been amicable, and opposition transformed into antagonism.

In a way it was understandable. Like the ancient Hebrews, Republicans had been in the desert for forty years, not a pleasant experience. Now it was time to repay the slights and rejections and condescension they had suffered, and Gingrich used his powers as speaker to unleash the pent-up emotions and bring new anger to bear. Confrontation was now the order of the day.

That was a special problem for AMHPS, which had predicated its strategy on appealing to both parties. "There was a period of craziness in the House," AMHPS lobbyist Dale Dirks recalled. "Newt Gingrich wasn't the only one carrying the Contract with America banner. It was many of the new Republicans that had been elected in that cycle and a lot of the existing Republicans who felt like they had had enough. . . . [I]t was pretty rough."[3]

AMHPS had grown comfortable with the way things were, with Stokes's office collaborating on legislation, with bills gathering support from Republicans as well as Democrats, with powerful Republicans joining ranks with Democrats to sweep aside what little opposition may have poked its head up. But now Stokes was in the minority, and his old cross-the-aisle relationships had largely frozen up. It was harder even for lobbyists to reach out to the other side. In the new congress, bipartisanship seemed an antique idea whose time was past and gone, unlamented, at least for those whom Gingrich's revolution had brought to power. "In that atmosphere," Dirks said, "it was an accomplishment just to stay alive."[4]

~

In the flush of the Republicans' unexpected victory, what Dirks and others saw as "the craziness" took hold of the legislative process. But unused to wielding power, the Republican fervor to root out the old and bring in radical changes stumbled on some of the realities of institutional life. Having been out in the wilderness for so long, the new majority had little idea of how the levers of governing actually worked. The Gingrichites fired everyone in the Office of House Legislative Counsel, which provided nonpartisan drafting services. Two weeks later, finding they had no one who knew how to write legislation, they had to hire them all back. Some of the new committee chairs, so initially swept up in the ideological fervor, began to drift back to their former belief in regular order and legislative proprieties.

Livingston, who had made such a memorable display of his cutlery, began to revert to his old institutional instincts and act as a traditional conservative chair, more in the manner of Bob Dole than of Gingrich. Porter, at the helm of the Labor H committee, was very much a moderate Republican, and a traditionalist. He had to sign Gingrich's oath, and he was under great pressure from the new radical crowd. But after the fever died back a bit, he began standing up to the populist tide, nowhere more apparent than in his commitment to health care.

Under the previous chair, William Natcher, the Labor H subcommittee had kept a fairly tight lid on partisanship, which was not difficult since Democrats seemed to be sitting permanently in the driver's seat. Natcher was cordial and frequently sought Republican agreement on funding issues, and while Republicans might complain and argue, the urgency just wasn't there. They weren't in power, and it seemed as if they never would be. Their opinions might gain a hearing, but they were not going to prevail.

As ranking member, Porter had his priorities—he was founder of the Congressional Human Rights Caucus—but they weren't controversial; and given the circumstances, he often spent time tending to other affairs. But when he took over as chair, he was suddenly all business. The committee's Republicans included middle-of-the-road moderates like himself, instinctively trying to maintain a modicum of normality, but also a fair share of bomb-throwers bent on doing away forever with business as usual. There was also a "Know Nothing" element, a presence of the populist extreme, slamming what they saw as silly and irrelevant medical science research at CDC and NIH.

Porter's job was especially challenging given that the Labor H bill included expenditures on issues the right hated, often dealing with sex: family planning and contraception, fetal tissue research, and abortion. Also, gun violence seen as a health issue. His first reflex was to buckle under the pressure Gingrich was bringing to bear, and the first Labor H bill was draconian. But as time passed, Porter began to fight back against Gingrich's scorched-earth zealots, ducking and weaving when he had to, acquiescing when it was necessary, but asserting himself when it came to his bed-rock principles. That was especially so when it came to medical science and health care.

Porter represented Illinois's 10th district, which was home to Northwestern University, with its Feinberg School of Medicine, a world-renowned medical school and research institute; his district also included a concentration of international pharmaceutical and biomedical companies—Baxter, Walgreens, Abbot Laboratories, and others. The 10th district was a focal point of medical science research and health-related enterprises. These were Porter's constituents. What he privately thought of the "Know Nothings" and the budget-slashing bomb-throwers doesn't have to be imagined. When he retired at age sixty-five, seven years after the Republican House revolution, he declared that the partisanship "had become so brutal and mindless that it was appalling."[5]

As Gingrich began to lose his grip, Porter came fully into his own as a leading advocate for medical research. (Porter's advocacy for health funding was so instrumental that NIH named a building for him, a rare honor.) Part of that was his protective stance regarding the Black health schools. His colleague in the

Senate in this endeavor was Arlen Specter, the Pennsylvania Republican who had partnered with Stokes on much of the AMHPS-inspired legislation. So even while the post-1994 political climate asphyxiated more than a few social welfare programs, AMHPS had a degree of shelter from the storm. The times weren't amenable to pursuing new legislative initiatives, but the funding for what already existed managed to survive intact.

Even Gingrich himself served as a partial shield, despite his fiery fiscal rhetoric. He might have been the irascible head of a pitchfork army, but he himself was a complex character. The charismatic leader of a Republican hard-right revolution, Gingrich was at the same time part academic intellectual and part traditional politician, who by 1994 had served eight terms, most of them as a more-or-less obscure back-bencher. Moreover, the scope of his intellectual curiosity was expansive, from American history to political theory to science, including medical science. At one point Porter brought a group of biotechnology experts to see Gingrich, and he engaged enthusiastically with their ideas. He had a special interest in NIH, especially in the translation of medical discoveries into practical use. Moreover, his respect for Morehouse School of Medicine and other Black medical institutions went back many years, as did his relationship with Sullivan, who had returned to the Morehouse presidency once his tenure as secretary was ended by Clinton's victory in 1992.

~

As the need for legislation on important national issues built, some of the right wing militance began to leak away, especially in the wake of two Gingrich-Clinton budget standoffs that precipitated government shutdowns. At the same time, Gingrich's effectiveness as a legislative manipulator slipped, which badly eroded the party's confidence in him. As his standing plummeted, a scandal concerning a long-time affair with a much younger congressional aide brought to light moral failures that pushed his tenure as speaker over the edge and into the abyss. By 1998 he had been driven out of the speakership. Shortly afterward he left Congress for good, declaring that he wasn't "willing to preside over people who are cannibals."[6]

As the Gingrich era careened toward its fiery end, AMHPS and its schools began to glimpse daylight. It was Senator Arlen Specter who provided the opportunity for their next big push.

A Pennsylvania Republican, Specter was one of Stokes's staunchest Senate allies. He had sponsored or cosponsored minority health legislation and was attuned to the needs of the AMHPS institutions and to the work of John Ruffin and his Office of Research on Minority Health. A great supporter of NIH (along with Porter), Specter had followed Ruffin's rocky journey at the Institutes, in particular his lack of funding and his need to plead for cooperation from often uninterested institute directors.

When in 1999 the Institute of Medicine (IOM) issued a report documenting the miniscule expenditures the National Cancer Institute was making on research specific to minorities, Specter seized on it to launch hearings in his appropriations subcommittee. Black women's death rates from breast cancer were higher than white women's. Prostate cancer rates in Black men were higher than in white men. Cervical cancer was more prevalent in Hispanic Americans than in white Americans. Asian Americans developed more stomach and liver cancers than white Americans. No one knew the reasons for these discrepancies—genetic, environmental, nutritional, vulnerability to viruses, or some other causes. As a result, no one knew what kinds of treatments might be most effective.

Little was known, and little was being done to find out. The National Cancer Institute in 1998 received $2.5 billion for research, of which only $24 *million* was spent specifically on minority disease, that is, less than 1 percent of the institute's budget. Richard Klausner, NCI's director, disputed that, saying that in fact $124 million was directed toward research on minorities, not $24 million. Most of this, though, was for more generally applicable studies that *indirectly* rather than *specifically* benefited minorities. A budget of $124 million would have been approximately 5 percent of the institute's budget. The National Cancer Institute enjoyed wide esteem, but the report rang a sour note of racial blindness.

Alfred Haynes had chaired the IOM committee that examined the National Cancer Institute funding. Haynes was president emeritus of the Charles Drew School of Medicine and one of the four original AMHPS institution leaders who had gone to see Margaret Heckler in 1983. He testified in front of Specter's committee, as did Klausner, as did Sullivan, whom Specter had invited as former HHS secretary.

Sullivan brushed aside Klausner's defense of his institute's allocation of resources. "What is needed," he said, "is an exponential leap forward in the orientation of NIH officials with respect to their approach to ethnic minorities and underserved communities."[7] That effort, he said, should be led by the Office of Research on Minority Health. That office, Sullivan told Specter's committee, needs to be elevated to a center, with a budget that will enable it to make its own grants—without having to go through other institutes. In a follow-up memo Sullivan underlined the funding deficiencies and the institutional indifference that so limited and frustrated Ruffin's efforts. He emphasized the urgency of addressing the problems of minority illness and disparities in care—starting by giving minority health its own center and its own funding.

In Specter, Sullivan had a more than willing audience. The Pennsylvania senator had been following the discussions about creating a minority health and health disparities center for several years, ever since AMHPS had raised the subject as a priority. The AMHPS board had focused on this, and Dirks and Ronny Lancaster, AMHPS's then president, had begun lobbying around the issue.

Sullivan had brought Lancaster to Washington as principal deputy assistant secretary. When Sullivan went back to Morehouse School of Medicine, Lancaster had gone with him as Morehouse's vice president for management and policy. With his hands full taking back the reins at the medical school, Sullivan had asked Lancaster to represent the school as its AMHPS board delegate; in 1997 Lancaster had been elected the association's president.

As AMHPS developed its effort to elevate Ruffin's office, Lancaster was in Washington almost every week, making rounds on the Hill, along with Dirks, informing, persuading, gathering support, bringing a proactive level of energy to the organization that had mostly been in a defensive huddle after the Gingrich revolution.

Lancaster was motivated. He was a young forty-two when he joined AMHPS. He had a master's degree from The Wharton School in health care policy and a law degree from Georgetown, where he specialized in health-related law. He had worked for former secretary Joseph Califano at HHS and had been a senior lobbyist for Blue Cross. He had been with Sullivan at the department for four years. Previous AMHPS presidents had been senior medical people immersed in the challenges of running hard-pressed institutions. Lancaster had the bandwidth they didn't, along with a skill set and knowledge base honed for his AMHPS role. He had a light but effective personal touch. The AMHPS presidents and deans recognized his assets and asked him to serve for repeated terms, breaking the rotation norm that had been in place since the organization's founding. Lancaster brought with him a strong work ethic, nor did he lack for ideas.

One day in March 1999, Lancaster was mulling over AMHPS's achievements—the research funding, the institutional funding, the centers of excellence funding, the scholarships and faculty loan waivers, the internship and training programs for young minority hopefuls—all of it working together to firm up the schools' financial health and broaden their scope as educational institutions. And yet, he thought, they are still fragile, still choked by their lack of resources, on shaky ground if real trouble were to hit. They had barely dodged the bullet when Gingrich's first budget went after their funding. There was hardly a school among them, he thought, that could survive a crisis.

What would it take, Lancaster thought, to give the schools the wherewithal to withstand earthquakes like that? Harvard's endowment then was more than $19 billion; Stanford's was over $9 billion. Meharry was hardly Harvard or Stanford, but still. Meharry's endowment was a blip, $2 million, a barely noticeable smudge on a balance sheet. And this for a school that had been in existence for over a hundred years. Morehouse's endowment was $3 million; Charles Drew's was less than $1 million; the other schools' endowments were less than that. These schools had all they could do to meet their current obligations. If you're struggling to pay ongoing bills, Lancaster thought, how do you put money aside to help insure your survivability?

It seemed improbable that any kind of legislation could address this issue, but Lancaster talked to Dirks about it. "What would you think," he said, "about creating a program whose sole purpose would be to give endowments to our schools, to give them some financial stability?" Dirks thought it was an idea worth pursuing.

With that encouragement, Lancaster approached Sullivan, who told him that something like an endowment act "didn't have a chance in hell of passing. But if you want to explore it," Sullivan said, "go right ahead."

As Lancaster and Dirks considered how such legislation might work, the obvious question loomed: How could enough members of Congress be persuaded to vote for a bill that would provide endowments for a select handful of schools? The obvious answer was that it couldn't happen. But what if a funding mechanism was already available that could support such a thing? None of the AMHPS-inspired legislation already in place could be used to generate endowment money—an enterprise of that sort wasn't within their purview. Could some kind of new enabling act draw sufficient support—which could then be used to fund endowments?

There in fact was already a statutory authority in place that was directing money to Black institutions—Ruffin's Office of Research on Minority Health. But Ruffin's office needed to find willing institutional partners in order to carry out projects. There were problems enough getting *any* minority-oriented research approved; proposals about endowments would be utterly out of the question. But, what if Ruffin's office was elevated to a center, with its own grantmaking power? In that case, money for endowments could be folded in, through the center's ordinary funding procedures. Raising the office to a center would give it the authority to support an endowment program.

With that in mind, Dirks went to the Office of House Legislative Counsel and had them draft a bill that would accomplish that objective. The bill they drafted—The Minority Health and Health Disparities Research and Education Act—established a "National Center on Minority Health and Health Disparities." One of this National Center's purposes would be "endowments," available to qualifying institutions that "do not have endowments that are worth in excess of an amount equal to 50 percent of the national average of endowment funds at institutions that conduct similar biomedical research or training of health professionals." None of

the AMHPS schools had any trouble meeting that particular qual-
ification. The Act (Public Act 106-525) authorized the appropriation committees to fund up to $100 million for the first year and
"such sums as may be necessary" for succeeding years.

~

With a draft bill now in hand, Lancaster and Dirks escalated their
lobbying campaign, bringing in some of AMHPS's major players:
David Satcher, who was now serving simultaneously as surgeon
general and assistant secretary of Health and Human Services;
Sullivan; Norman Francis; John Maupin, president of Meharry;
and National Medical Association president Gary Dennis, a Howard Medical School neurosurgeon whose testimony in front of
several committees was especially effective.

Starting off with Atlanta congressman John Lewis, Dirks and
Lancaster reached out to the geographical constituencies that
always allowed AMHPS to punch above its weight—the representatives from Alabama, Georgia, Louisiana, Tennessee, Texas,
California, and Florida, where the AMHPS schools were located.
In Tennessee, Meharry president Maupin had developed a good
relationship with Senator Bill Frist, a rising force in Republican
politics. Frist was a Nashville-born transplant surgeon, a professor at Vanderbilt Medical School, and the first physician to serve in
the Senate for many decades. Elected in the Republican sweep
in 1994, Frist was the party's deputy whip and would soon be
elected majority leader.

A stalwart conservative on many issues, Frist was at the same
time a leading advocate for health care and a supporter of Meharry
and the other Black medical institutions. Satcher had known Frist
and his family since Satcher was inaugurated as Meharry's president in 1982 (Frist's parents had given Satcher a check for $250,000
then, an indication of their belief in the school, which was at that
point fighting for its life). Frist himself had attended Maupin's in-

auguration as Meharry's president in 1994, and the two men had developed a warm friendship. Satcher and Maupin enlisted Frist's help with the bill, and he became essential in generating Republican support in the Senate, signing on to sponsor the bill along with Ted Kennedy.

In the House the AMHPS lobbying effort had no trouble finding sponsors among Democrats, and within a short period, eighty representatives had signed on. By this time Stokes had retired after serving thirty years in one of the House's most storied careers. His place on the House Appropriations Committee had been taken by Jesse Jackson Jr., a Democrat from Illinois, who became the bill's lead sponsor. Jackson was chafing at the bit to introduce the bill, but it was painfully clear to everyone that a bill with eighty Democratic sponsors and zero Republicans would be going nowhere in a Republican-controlled legislature. Introducing the bill under those circumstances would kill it in its cradle and destroy hopes for bringing minority issues to the fore at NIH.

Casting around for a strategy, Lancaster and Dirks decided to visit Charlie Norwood, the Republican representative from Georgia's 10th district. Norwood, like Bill Frist, had come in as part of the 1994 Republican sweep, running on his support for Gingrich's Contract with America. On most issues he was a hard-nosed, blunt-spoken conservative. He argued for tight controls on immigration and advocated sending a forty-thousand-man military force to guard the Mexican border. Later in his career he voted against renewing the Voting Rights Act, declaring that it discriminated against Southern states over practices that were long past. At the same time, Lancaster and Dirks knew Norwood had a strong record on health care; he had been a dentist before going into politics, and he remained actively involved in dental and other health issues. Beyond that, in 1996 Norwood's district had been redrawn, and he now had a far larger number of African American

constituents than he had had previously. Given those circumstances, Norwood, they thought, might possibly be persuaded to
join the bill.

When they went to see him, Norwood wasn't in his office, but
his legislative assistant, Rodney Whitlock, told them, "I've talked
to Mr. Norwood about this. He is 100 percent behind this bill." The
bill, with eighty Democrats and one Republican, was now "bipartisan," which was how Jackson and the Congressional Black Caucus's Donna Christensen introduced it at a press conference two
days later.

Charlie Norwood's name on the bill was the key. It allowed
Dirks and Lancaster to present it as bipartisan, which to most
people meant that it had the support of numbers of Republicans
as well as Democrats. Those with any level of understanding knew
there was only one Republican sponsor, but Norwood's courage
in putting his name forward made it possible for Dirks and Lancaster to successfully lobby other Republicans. Jackson's role in
this was key. He had taken Stokes's place on the Labor H committee and he had inherited Stokes's bipartisan approach as well.
His outreach to Norwood was critical, and Jackson, Dirks, and
Lancaster worked nonstop to attract additional Republican
support.

Those they approached included J. C. Watts, who chaired the
House Republican Leadership Conference. Watts was one of only
two Black House Republicans. Like Norwood, he was an aggres-
sive fiscal conservative, but he was also a strong supporter of the
Black educational institutions. Norwood and Watts pushed the
bill. Together they were a persuasive force, hard for their fellow
Republicans to ignore, and so the act to establish a National Center on Minority Health and Health Disparities actually moved forward on a strong bipartisan basis. When the bill was eventually

considered on the House floor, it was Norwood who managed its passage.

~

In both the House and Senate, the bill was gaining momentum, but there was one major roadblock—the NIH itself. NIH director Harold Varmus was adamantly opposed.

Varmus was one of the world's most distinguished scientists. A Nobel laureate, he had won the prize in 1989 (along with Michael Bishop) for his work on how cellular gene mutations, so-called oncogenes, lead to cancer. In 1993 he was appointed by President Clinton as NIH director, succeeding Bernadine Healy.

Varmus had graduated from Columbia as a physician but had made a life in the laboratory rather than at the bedside, doing research into the basic functions of cells and viruses. He had brought his researcher's worldview with him as NIH director, which meant, among other things, that he believed decisions about the allocation of resources should be made strictly on the basis of the merits of research proposals as measured against other research proposals. From the beginning of his tenure he wasn't happy with the idea of an office, let alone a center, devoted to minority health and health disparities. How was that basic science? He questioned the legitimacy of it. The incidence of disease among minorities, he believed, was not relevant to NIH's mission; besides which, many of the NIH institutes were doing work beneficial to minorities, and therefore that was not a real problem.

Sullivan begged to differ. As one of the leading advocates for the center, and with the weight of his former office (in which he had overseen NIH), Sullivan was able to meet with Varmus several times. The meetings were not always cordial. In one heated discussion, Varmus declared that before he'd allow Ruffin's office to become a center, he'd lay down in the middle of Wisconsin

Avenue. To which Sullivan replied that he didn't think that would be such a good idea; he could get rolled over.

Varmus's thoughts on the subject were in a way typical of the era. It had only been a few years earlier when women were rarely included in disease studies. They weren't considered necessary, said one critic; the research community essentially looked at them medically as if they were just smaller men. But Healy, Varmus's predecessor as director, had launched the Women's Health Initiative, a large, longitudinal study of postmenopausal women's health, and she had pushed for women's general inclusion in clinical trials. NIH had bowed to the pressure and had created policy changes, encouraging the enrollment of women in trials; but it had been slow in adhering to its own guidelines, so much so that Congress had passed a law mandating it. That kind of exclusionary psychology was still firmly in place regarding minorities. No separate attention was necessary since minorities were only slightly different versions of white people. Few ever thought to look at minority health as a field with its own distinct characteristics.

Varmus was an imposing figure, intimidating to most of the institute directors and to anyone else who might oppose him. Although distinctly unsympathetic to the center idea, he was open to discussion. His talks with Sullivan did not go well, nor did a meeting with Ronny Lancaster and Howard College of Medicine neurosurgeon Gary Dennis, then president of the National Medical Association.

The meeting took place in the director's conference room in NIH's Building One. At the table, Lancaster sat on one side of Varmus and Dennis sat on the other. Around the room's periphery were NIH institute directors or their deputies, plus Dirks and Ruffin, whose office was at issue. The meeting started off with Lancaster and Dennis explaining to Varmus why the legislation was so badly needed and why they were going to make it happen if they possibly could. They were there to ask him to consider that and to ask if he could not see a way to support the bill.

Varmus was not moved. At one point he addressed Dennis by his first name, "Gary," a breach of etiquette in meetings like this where participants always referred to each other as "doctor." Lancaster was attuned to this more than others; he was the only "mister" in the room. When Varmus said, "Gary," Dennis responded, "Well, Harold . . ." To Lancaster, all the directors seemed frozen in shock. But after that, he considered that he, too, was on a first-name basis with the intimidating Dr. Varmus, and from then on, the meeting was among Harold, Gary, and Ronny.

To buttress their argument, Lancaster and Dennis had brought along an issue of *The Chronicle of Higher Education*, which had published an article on NIH funding for minority scientists. According to the NIH's own data, less than 0.5 percent of total grant dollars was going to African American investigators, 0.6 percent was going to Asian American investigators, and 0.7 percent to Hispanic investigators; in aggregate, less than 2 percent of NIH's medical science money was being awarded to minority scientists.

Those numbers caught everyone's attention. They cast a glaring light on NIH's utter failure to support minority scientists and institutions. Lancaster and Dennis explained how lack of research support for minority training and medical science institutions meant fewer minority physicians and scientists, which constricted minority access to health care and impeded the understanding of disease among minorities, which contributed to the dire state of minority health. They connected the dots. Against these arguments, Varmus's objections became less and less tenable. It was not a good meeting for him.

Shortly afterwards, HHS Secretary Donna Shalala called Satcher, her assistant secretary, and told him that unless Varmus came on board, the department wouldn't be able to support the legislation, which meant that the administration would withhold its support, which meant the bill would go nowhere. With that, Satcher talked with Varmus, who invited him to his monthly meeting with the NIH institute directors.

When Satcher started his presentation, he sensed he was in front of a negative audience. But he laid out his argument in his usual courteous style, which seemed to naturally embrace his listeners. By the time he finished, the tension had lifted and the questioning—from both Varmus and his directors—went on in an atmosphere more friendly than not. Satcher later recalled it as being one of the more memorable meetings of his time in government.

Varmus made no commitments at the meeting. But a week later, he sent a strong letter of support to Shalala. Satcher never knew what the most significant factor in Varmus's change of mind might have been. Most likely it was the accumulation of documentation and arguments that induced him to reexamine his preconceptions, which spoke to an open mind, even in the face of his own strong, long-held opinions. When Varmus left the directorship, Ruffin, his adversary for years, gave him a lifetime achievement award. (It's worth noting that Varmus is currently overseeing a New York Genome Center project aimed at understanding racial disparities in the prevalence of various types of cancers.)

With both Republican and Democrat support in Congress and the administration's strong backing now that Varmus had changed his mind, the bill was fast-tracking its way through the markups and onto the floor of both chambers. The hope was to get the bill through quickly. It was already mid-October. The 2000 presidential election was only a few weeks off. Al Gore and George W. Bush were locked in a tight race, and members of Congress were at critical junctures in their own campaigns.

At the last moment AMHPS learned that an unnamed Republican senator had put the bill on "hold," a procedure that allows a senator to prevent a bill from coming to a vote. Word got to AMHPS that this senator was not opposed to the bill as such, but that he had issues with Senator Frist. Frist was sponsoring the bill along with Ted Kennedy, and holding up this bill put Frist on notice that the senator was determined to get his problem heard and resolved. Dirks and Lancaster knew that if the bill was derailed now, it might well be killed altogether. A new president, with a new and rearranged Congress, could spell unpredictable difficulties. The support was lined up right now, after years of work. The upcoming election was a potential disaster.

With tension building among the AMHPS leaders, they tried to reach out to Frist. But he was nowhere to be found. Finally, Meharry president John Maupin managed to track him down through Frist's chief of staff—he was in Chattanooga at a fund-raiser.

When Frist heard what had happened, he flew back to Washington and took care of the problem. Neither Maupin nor anyone else at AMHPS knew what transpired between Frist and his unhappy colleague, but to their vast relief the hold was released. The bill went back onto the docket and proceeded toward a vote.

On November 22, 2000, the day before Thanksgiving, President Clinton signed the bill into law. It had been a close call in the House, where it passed by one vote, but in the Senate the vote was unanimous. It was the last bill President Clinton (already a lame duck) signed. With House Labor H Committee chair Porter behind it and Arlen Specter chairing the Senate appropriations subcommittee, funding was more or less guaranteed. The number for the first year came in at $80 million.

$\sim$

The Minority Health and Health Disparities Research and Education Act, initiated by Lancaster and Dirks, was brought to fruition through the committed support of many members of Congress: in the House, Democrats Jessie Jackson Jr., William Clay,

Donna Christensen, and many others, Republicans Charlie Norwood and J. C. Watts. In the Senate, Arlen Specter, Bill Frist, Tom Harkin, and Ted Kennedy played important roles. But AMHPS did the heavy lifting throughout, and over time the Act brought very considerable benefits to the AMHPS institutions. The sense of satisfaction and triumph among those clustered around the *Resolute* desk when President Clinton signed the bill into law was palpable.

But the Act was complex; its mechanisms had to be mastered before they could bolster the schools as they were intended to do; and the acceptance of health disparities as a legitimate research topic was still questionable across the NIH centers and institutes.

But AMHPS had a platform now. The question was, How were they going to use it? AMHPS was almost a quarter century old; its founding generation—Sullivan, Satcher, Walter Bowie, Alfred Haynes, Lloyd Elam, Tony Rachal, Norman Francis—were heavily involved elsewise, moving toward retirement, even passing from the scene. Stokes, whose dynamic leadership had given the legislative charge its energy, had gone back home to practice law and to teach. A new leadership was coming to the fore in the minority health professions schools. It wasn't clear what their agenda might be, or how they might try to carry it out.

CHAPTER 10

A National Institute

AMHPS faced the millennial year with great expectations. A Republican, George W. Bush, was now in the White House, which might have suggested less money for social programs and less engagement with minority concerns. But the AMHPS schools had done well under previous Republican administrations. Much of the pillar legislation had been established during Ronald Reagan's presidency, and George H. W. Bush had appointed Louis Sullivan HHS secretary, with all the positive impetus to the association. Even during the dark Gingrich days, AMHPS had managed to hold its own.

From its beginning the association had worked a bipartisan strategy, and the campaign for the National Center had proven its effectiveness. Power players in both parties, in both chambers, had rallied to pass the enabling act in 2000, and Republican-led appropriations committees in the House and Senate had funded the act liberally. The elation spurred by the elevation of John Ruffin's office to a center was not just for the immense victory it represented but for a future that carried with it good hope that the minority institutions would continue to get stronger and that the government would confront disparate health care with increasing vigor.

Those were not pie-in-the-sky hopes. Public Law 106-525, the Minority Health and Health Disparities Research and Education Act of 2000, which established the National Center on Health and Health Disparities, had gotten its start when Ronny Lancaster was caught up by the idea that the viability of the fragile minority health institutions would be enhanced, perhaps even dependent on developing some halfway reasonable endowments instead of the threadbare backup sums in their current accounts. Elevating Ruffin's Office of Research on Minority Health into an NIH center was, Lancaster and Dale Dirks believed, the vehicle for making that happen.

Ruffin's office was, of course, an NIH entity, and NIH was a medical research institution, so the endowment provisions needed to be focused on research. In the act, they were termed "research endowments" (in contrast to general endowments)—funds that would enable the AMHPS and other minority-oriented health schools to create long-term resources that would support their research-related endeavors. A research endowment program would provide a level of support for recipient institutions that would enable them to build a significant bank of resources they wouldn't need not consume, a sum that would accrue on a yearly basis and would be enlarged by interest and investment. (In contrast, federal grants ordinarily need to be used within the time period fixed by the grant, commonly one fiscal year. At the end of the grant term, the expectation is that all the funds will have been spent on the research project, leaving nothing in the account. The researcher would have started with zero and ended with zero, with nothing left over that could be used as a reserve.)

Dirks, Lancaster, and their colleagues knew that a center would be a major accomplishment, a huge breakthrough. And now they had successfully got it through Congress.

This was monumentally significant in terms of empowering medical research at AMHPS and AMHPS-like institutions and strengthening their overall fiscal health. From today's perspective, the results of twenty years of the endowment program have proved the concept. Research resources at recipient schools have built up dramatically, as have reserve accounts. The endowment funds at Morehouse and Meharry in 2020 are above $100 million each, still negligible next to Harvard's $41 billion or Stanford's $28 billion, but they are more than thirty times larger than what they had been.

In addition, the National Center Act gave Ruffin a budget—$80 million that first year—plus it gave him the ability to award grants himself instead of going around "with a tin cup in his hand," as one observer put it, to other NIH centers and institutes. Having his own money changed his relationship to other NIH entities. He was now not only able to award his own grants, he also had financial leverage to attract collaborations with other centers and institutes on minority health projects that before this would have gone begging.

In addition to the provision of granting research endowments, the act had picked up three other key provisions as it made its way through the lobbying process and committee debates. These three other key provisions were: a "centers of excellence" program (where the Center could designate specific schools as leaders in minority health and health care disparities); a loan repayment program; and a mandate to create and implement an NIH-wide strategic plan on health care disparities. Together these three and the endowment provision constituted what might be thought of as an

NIH health disparities core infrastructure. Previous minority health legislation had addressed one or more needs of the minority health professions schools and had been administered by various agencies. This act concentrated a series of key measures to aggressively address the problem of inequitable health care under the aegis of the National Institutes of Health.

～

The very first modern assertion of America's obligation to care for the health of its Black and other minority populations had been posited in 1985 by Margaret Heckler in her now famous report and in her appointment of an HHS deputy assistant secretary for minority health. That modest beginning had now broadened into a core element of the National Institutes of Health, the nation's premier medical science research institution. The evolution had taken a quarter of a century.

The sense of accomplishment generated by the passage of the National Center Act in 2000 was immensely gratifying for the AMHPS leaders who had precipitated it and seen it through. The act lifted their optimism as they looked toward the future. No doubt it reminded those with a historical bent of the time frames involved in moving the nation forward. Health inequity was a persistent, hard-to-address reality, embedded as normal in American health care and health care systems. It did not and would not yield ground easily. But meanwhile, the National Center Act provided important tools to attack the problem, and Ruffin, with advice from his advisors, was figuring out how to most effectively use them.

Along with research endowments, the act established a loan repayment program and a "centers of excellence" program. The NIH category "center of excellence" originated many decades earlier, and it had become a common NIH funding mechanism. "Centers of excellence" designated certain institutions as leaders in the study of a particular field of disease and the implementation of developments in that field. There are centers of excellence in Alzheimer's disease, muscular dystrophy, geriatric medicine, and in many other fields—essentially in all the medical and developmental areas represented by the NIH's institutes and centers.

These centers of excellence—institutions that had established themselves as key to progress in their fields—were eligible to receive a special category of large grants focused on their particular specialty. These grants were meant to stimulate research, foster collaborations, and provide career-building opportunities for postdoctoral fellows, junior faculty, and early-stage researchers. They were intended, among other objectives, to attract and train younger research scientists working in a particular field—in this case minority health and health disparities.

AMHPS's argument here was that many mainstream institutions were being rewarded for their role in fields such as neuroscience, cancer, and heart disease. Progress in these disciplines was considered essential to public health. Likewise, understanding minority health and health disparities was also crucial; progress here was no less essential to public health. If Johns Hopkins University and the University of Pennsylvania were being accorded funding as centers of excellence in their particular specialties, so should leading institutions in the study of minority disease and disparate care.

The first institutions to receive a center of excellence designation under the National Center on Minority Health and Health Disparities included Drew, Howard, Morehouse, Tuskegee, and Meharry. The designations gave new attention to minority health and allowed Ruffin to funnel money into studies focused on understanding and ameliorating minority morbidity and mortality, which were so markedly divergent from mainstream levels of disease and death. This in the face of continued deep-seated skepticism within

NIH's medical science community about the very validity of the subject. Funding from the centers of excellence program helped further stabilize the AMHPS institutions financially at the same time as it expanded their research programs and increased their ability to attract more Black research scientists.

~

The act's third key provision, the loan repayment program, furthered the recruitment and support of young Black PhD scientists by providing educational loan repayments of up to $35,000 a year in return for recipients committing to conduct two years of health disparities or clinical research. Since 50 percent of these loan recipients were mandated to come from disadvantaged backgrounds, the loan repayment program increased economic diversity among the emerging cohort of Black medical scientists. The loan repayment program was a success from its launch in 2001, averaging over 250 awards per year out of some 600 applicants. David Satcher saw that the AMHPS schools had been able to recruit "in a short period of time an unbelievable army of people interested in the elimination of health disparities."[1] That may have been a bit of an overstatement, but the pipeline was certainly beginning to fill up.

It wasn't only the historically Black schools that benefited from the loan repayment and centers of excellence programs. As the bill was moving forward in the upper chamber, Senator Robert Byrd, Democrat of West Virginia, introduced an additional factor into the discussion. Byrd said he understood the importance of racial and ethnic minority issues in health care, but there were other nonminority populations equally underserved and equally in need. Parts of West Virginia were entrenched in multigenerational poverty. Uninsured or inadequately insured, often with limited access to physicians, a large number of Byrd's constituents presented the same acute health problems as poor Blacks and other

minorities. Why, he asked, should impoverished white populations not be included in the act's provisions?

In 2000, Byrd was eighty-three years old, and he had at that
point served in the Senate for forty-one years. He had been both
majority and minority leader; he was the senior Democrat on the
Appropriations Committee, which he had chaired various times.
He was president pro tempore of the Senate, third in the line of
presidential succession. Byrd's support for the bill could not be
jeopardized, besides which, AMHPS was not opposed to the point
he was making about impoverished white populations. As a result,
the final bill included language that incorporated Byrd's concerns.
"The general purpose of the National Center on Minority Health
and Health Disparities," the act read, "is the conduct and support
of research, training, dissemination of information, and other programs with respect to minority health conditions *and other populations with health disparities*" (emphasis added). Those "other
populations" were the sociologically disadvantaged and underserved rural populations of West Virginia and other Appalachian
states.

In its "Findings" section, the act states, "The largest number
of the medically underserved are white individuals, and many of
them have the same healthcare access problems as do members
of minority groups. Nearly 20,000,000 white individuals live be-
low the poverty line with many living in nonmetropolitan, rural
areas such as Appalachia, where the high percentage of counties
designated as health professional shortage areas (47 percent) and
the high rate of poverty contribute to disparity outcomes."

The inclusion of underserved white populations in a bill initiated by historically Black schools in order to strengthen predominantly Black institutions suggests a phenomenon whose dynamic
we have seen before. AMHPS's founding document, authored by
Ruth Hanft, *Blacks and the Health Professions in the '80s* had

precipitated Margaret Heckler's *Report of the Secretary's Task Force on Black and Minority Health.* In the transmutation of the AMHPS white paper into the Heckler Report, Black concerns had expanded into Black *and minority* concerns. The same had happened in 1987 with the Excellence in Minority Health Education and Care Act. Narrowly drafted to benefit four historically Black institutions— Meharry Medical College, Meharry School of Dentistry, Xavier University College of Pharmacy, and Tuskegee School of Veterinary Medicine—that act had soon folded in the other AMHPS schools and also Hispanic-serving and Native American–serving institutions. Now, the NIH Office of Research on Minority Health had become a Center whose purpose was to benefit poor whites as well as ethnic and racial minorities. In these instances, it's possible to recognize the mostly unseen workings of the democratic ethos, almost inevitably spreading its penumbra over different groups of the society's marginalized and disregarded.

These were not just "words on parchment," inserted into the act for effect. The AMHPS leadership anticipated that institutions like the University of West Virginia Health System would be both interested and eligible. Institutions in West Virginia, Virginia, and Kentucky participated. As time passed, institutions in Alabama, Arkansas, New Mexico, Texas, and other states accessed these programs.

In reflecting on this phenomenon, John Maupin expressed how most of the AMHPS leaders felt. "AMHPS was an advocate for the African American community. We had a host of challenges beyond what others faced. But we were never saying that to anyone's exclusion. We wanted the rest of the country to understand that there are a lot of communities that are left out of available health care. We weren't the only population that was vulnerable. . . . We knew that if you listened to what we had to say, you could extrapolate that to the benefit to others, to the benefit of this country."[2]

There was no rhetorical fanfare about the equivalence and essential unity of minority and poor white populations in regard to health care and health disparities, but the act embodied that largely unremarked fact. Representing the constituents he represented for as long as he had represented them, Senator Byrd knew how true that was. When Arkansas public health director Dr. Joycelyn Elders (later surgeon general) had first visited the county health clinics in her state, she remarked that the health problems in the Mississippi Delta with its mostly Black population and the Ozarks with its mostly white population mirrored each other. "It was all the same," she said. "One was a like a photo negative of the other."[3]

~

The National Center Act's fourth key provision (in addition to research endowments, centers of excellence, and a loan repayment program) mandated that the new Center's director, Ruffin, create a comprehensive plan to support, conduct, and coordinate health disparities research across all of NIH's centers and institutes. That is, all NIH institutes and centers (such as the National Cancer Institute; the National Heart, Lung, and Blood Institute; and the National Asthma and Infectious Disease Institute) were to collaborate in an NIH-wide strategic plan for addressing health disparities—under Ruffin's leadership. This strategic plan was supposed to be in place within twelve months.

Here was a congressional declaration that the problem of health disparities was so deep and so embedded that the nation's premier medical research institution, across all its branches, was to conduct and support research to understand it and counter it. Ruffin was seized by this objective and its implications and moved quickly on this provision.

He did not meet with instant success, or much in the way of any success. The plan he submitted to Congress, with input from NIH director Elias Zerhouni (who had succeeded Harold Varmus), HHS secretary Tommy Thompson, and the Center's own advisory council, faced repeated delays. When he time and again asked the NIH institutes and centers to provide plans and budgets for their participation in the strategic plan, he met resistance. "This persistence," he wrote after he retired, "added fuel to the fire for those who already did not like the idea of having an NIH center dedicated to minority health issues."[4] Repeated iterations of the plan encountered one thorny problem after another, not least of which was defining which groups could legitimately qualify as health disparity populations. But by 2007 the Center had recognized women, veterans, prisoners, and LGBTQ individuals as qualifying populations.

Ruffin's intense frustration at the refusal of NIH to commit wholeheartedly to a cross-institute, large-scale assault on health disparities became obvious after he retired from the agency. "Laws," he wrote in his 2015 memoir *Going the Distance*, "are made to be implemented and enforced, not broken." And: "Minority health and health disparity issues [need to] remain a top priority at the agency . . . *a status [they have] yet to gain*" (emphasis added). This was written fifteen years after Ruffin began his campaign to mobilize NIH resources across the board. "It is not enough," he wrote, "to have an interest in minority health and health disparities. . . . A priority commands substantial investment of resources; in this case that would be dollars, people, and space. While the investment in minority health and health disparities research gradually has increased over the years, it remains at the low end of the funding priority scale for the agency."[5] In 2020, five years after Ruffin's remarks, the (now) Institute of Minority Health and Health Disparities has the second-lowest budget of the twenty-three NIH institutes—$335 million, less than 1 percent of NIH's total budget of $41.6 billion.

Dale Dirks, Ronny Lancaster, and John Maupin (who succeeded Lancaster as AMHPS president in 2003) were more intent on getting the research endowments, centers of excellence, and loan repayment program underway. These were substantive, immediate contributors to the financial well-being and research capacity of the AMHPS schools. The school presidents and deans wanted to financially strengthen their notoriously underfunded institutions and expand their footprints in the worlds of clinical medicine and medical science. To Dirks and his colleagues, a comprehensive, cross-NIH strategy was a complicated, long-term project, less urgent than the funding programs, more aspirational.

Ruffin didn't necessarily disagree, and he quickly got to work putting in place the mechanisms for letting and administering grants and loan repayments. But he persisted in his drive to mobilize a large-scale strategy. John Ruffin was engaged in the long fight.

~

In the scope of history, America's engagement with the health of Blacks and other people of color has been a recent phenomenon. The first post-Reconstruction formal recognition that there was a problem that needed attention didn't come until 1985. Thomas Malone, who chaired Margaret Heckler's Task Force on Black and Minority Health, had written about "the necessity for an accelerated national assault on the persistent health disparities." Health disparities, the Heckler Report said, were "a tragic dilemma," that required "efforts of monumental proportions." In case "monumental" efforts might have sounded hyperbolic, the Heckler Report documented in its first table that there were 58,942 excess Black deaths for the years 1979–1981, that is, Black deaths above and beyond what might have been expected if Blacks were dying at the same rate as other Americans.[6] The morbidity numbers were as shocking as the mortality statistics.

Every legislative act that AMHPS initiated was a further statement that the federal government recognized the problem. Every piece of legislation was a step toward addressing it. A comprehensive NIH strategy of the kind the National Center Act envisioned, and John Ruffin pursued so assiduously, would have been a leap in the direction of paying attention and taking action at scale.

To Ruffin's ongoing dissatisfaction, that did not happen. If it had, the level of awareness among NIH scientists and their extramural colleagues would have risen some degree; but even if that happened, the nation's 600,000 physicians (in 2000) would still have remained largely untouched by the knowledge, and the nation's 240 million white citizens would still have remained almost entirely oblivious. The severity of the health disparities problem, its profound consequences for Black lives, and its ramifications for the general population would still not have entered into the nation's consciousness.

Then in 2003 a bombshell exploded. The Institute of Medicine (IOM; now the National Academy of Medicine) published a hefty volume titled *Unequal Treatment: Confronting Racial and Ethnic Disparities in Healthcare*. IOM, the prestigious independent medical advisor to the government, one of the three National Academies (Science and Engineering are the other two), had been tasked by Congress to assess the problem of racial and ethnic health care disparities. A committee headed by Brian Smedley, an IOM senior program officer in the Division of Health Sciences Policy, brought together a great number of studies regarding biased and disparate care that had appeared in a variety of journals across the medical literature but that had never achieved a critical mass that drew attention. *Unequal Treatment* provided a comprehensive summary and synthesis of that scattered literature. Instead of the drip, drip,

drip of papers appearing here and there, over many years, here it all was, carefully reviewed, organized, and clarified for the broad audience of health care providers and medical scientists.

Unequal Treatment shocked the medical world. The book illuminated an underside of American health care that most doctors had no idea existed. Here we are, the book announced, at the beginning of the twenty-first century, four decades after the civil rights laws were passed, and the medical world is still riven with prejudice and discrimination.[7] The details were mostly known by those engaged with these things before *Unequal Treatment* was published. But even in that small world, the extent of inequitable care documented by Smedley and his committee of experts was startling.

Every medical specialty from cardiology to oncology to orthopedics to psychiatry and down the line had its own grim history of biased care. "Racial and ethnic disparities are found in a range of other disease [in addition to cardiovascular and cancer care] and health service categories, including diabetes care, end-stage renal disease and transplantation, pediatric care and maternal and child health, mental health, rehabilitative and nursing home services, and many surgical procedures."[8]

For Augustus White, Harvard chief of orthopedic surgery, it was the disparities in care of long bone fracture that stood out to him. "In my own field," he wrote, "just why in the world was it that African Americans brought into ERs with long bone fractures were less likely to receive opioids and other analgesics?"[9]

Unequal Treatment itself had its own interesting back story. Smedley, the study director and lead editor, was a PhD clinical psychologist who specialized in public health policy. He was at the time the only African American study director in IOM's Division of Health Sciences Policy. IOM was esteemed for the rigor and objectivity of its studies, a standard it maintained in large part through the makeup of its study committees. These study committees were composed of world-class scientists, some with clear but divergent points of view on questions, others with equally good credentials but who were perceived as more or less neutral on the subject at hand.

But racial prejudice in medicine was a volatile issue, sure to be controversial. The president of IOM at the time was Kenneth Shine, a distinguished cardiologist but not a political progressive. He was not eager for this committee to shine a spotlight on racism in medicine, and he took an active role in making sure there were committee members who were skeptical on the issue of racial disparities, as indeed was true of many in NIH and IOM circles. Shine named as chair of the committee Alan Nelson, past president of the AMA. Nelson, who practiced in Utah, had had little contact with African Americans either as patients or colleagues. But although Nelson might have begun his job as a skeptic, by the time the committee completed its work, he was livid about the disparities that existed and the human suffering that had been, and still was, being experienced by African Americans and other people of color.

The results documented in *Unequal Treatment* were not just devastating, they were incontrovertible. The volume became a playbook for AMHPS, as Maupin and Dirks pushed hard on the appropriation committee representatives and senators for continued funding. Just as Louis Stokes had used the Heckler Report to pressure witnesses and fellow committee members, AMHPS was now using *Unequal Treatment*, with its IOM imprimatur.

Unequal Treatment put forward a series of recommendations to help alleviate the destructive consequences of disparate care. One key strategy it advanced was to increase diversity among health care professionals. Minority practitioners were far more likely to establish themselves in medically underserved communities. But minority patients in all communities responded better to treatment by minority physicians; they adhered better to therapies, they expressed greater satisfaction, and their outcomes improved. The American population, *Unequal Treatment* noted, was growing in diversity and would continue on that trajectory. To serve that population, the country needed a more diverse body of health practitioners. Other recommendations were for more research "to identify sources of racial and ethnic disparities" and to understand the "barriers to eliminating disparities."

AMHPS had been driving those points home for years. A broad swath of Americans lacked adequate medical care. The deficiencies were glaring. Many of the reasons for disparities were opaque; they needed to be understood in order for disparities to be reduced or eliminated. The minority health professions schools were key in the effort to better these pictures. These were AMHPS's arguments precisely.

⁓

For fifteen years AMHPS-inspired legislation had been strengthening the schools, stabilizing their finances, building their faculties and student bodies, and expanding the scope of their research endeavors and clinical training. But where now did all this effort stand? What real-world consequences was it having?

A year or so after *Unequal Treatment* was published, another report came out examining just this question. The answer it gave was not encouraging. The report, *Missing Persons: Minorities in the Health Professions*, came about through a grant from the W. K. Kellogg Foundation to Duke University to explore the state of diversity in medicine and other health professions. Kellogg and several associated foundations—Josiah Macy and Robert Wood Johnson—were troubled by the numbers they were seeing regarding the lack of growth among minority health professionals. To get a clear understanding of the situation, they established a commission of sixteen people, including Louis Sullivan, who served as chairman. The sixteen members of Sullivan's commission included legal and business leaders, as well as medical experts. To make sure that whatever answers the commission came up with would gain political attention, Sullivan asked Bob Dole and retired congressman Paul Rogers to serve as honorary cochairs. Dole had been the long-term Republican Senate leader and had run for president against Bill Clinton. Rogers, a Democrat from Florida, had been known as "Mr. Health" for his health care advocacy.

To Sullivan and his commission, the stagnating numbers were alarming; they indicated that minorities' access to health care would worsen and that disparate care would become an even greater problem. They looked at the historical trendlines. In the 1950s, the number of Black physicians in the country was, relatively speaking, negligible. Meharry and Howard were together graduating about 200 medical doctors a year, the Northern medical schools a few more, the Southern schools none. The numbers had slowly increased in the 1960s, '70s and '80s when many new medical schools had come on line.

The civil rights movement had focused attention on issues of justice and equality, which had an effect on medical schools as well as the rest of society. Martin Luther King Jr.'s murder had jolted many institutions into examining their customary exclusion of Blacks; many had created deanships for diversity or minority affairs to help with the identification, recruitment, and retention of minority students. At Boston University a faculty committee including Sullivan, a professor there at the time, had received support from the dean and had approached the other New England medical schools with the idea of holding a recruitment weekend for African American students from historically Black colleges and universities, most of them in the South. The other schools had responded enthusiastically. All of the attending students had received acceptances, and the medical institutions had opened doors that historically had been mostly shut tight.[10]

So the numbers had risen, but not as robustly as many had anticipated. The surge of commitment to improving diversity conflicted with the heavy weight of custom and the still-prevalent (even if now somewhat muted) mindset that assumed Blacks were intellectually less than capable. Harvard Medical School was a prime case of the conflict between a desire to do better and an ingrained institutional racism. In the wake of the King assassination, Harvard's medical faculty debated the question of increasing the number of Black enrollees. A committee of professors argued that the number of Black students should be increased from the usual two or three a year to fifteen (in a class of 100). Those opposed responded that this itself would be a quota and was, therefore, unacceptable—a rationalization, many felt, for some deeper, unspoken resistance to the proposal; after all, Harvard had long operated on the basis of a severe quota *restricting* Black enrollment. A compromise was eventually reached. Harvard would take fifteen Black students each year, but the size of the class would be increased from 100 to 115, to counter the perception that "less qualified" Black students had displaced fifteen qualified white students.

The numbers of Black medical students and emerging doctors had continued to increase in the two decades following King's death, but by the end of the 1980s, minority physicians were still, as Sullivan told newly elected President George H. W. Bush, "grossly underrepresented." In the year 2004, it was clear that the trajectory in the numbers of emerging minority doctors had flattened out. This at the same time as the country's population was growing in diversity, a trend that was only going to speed up. "The U.S. medical profession is on a demographic collision course with an increasingly diverse nation," the Sullivan commission declared. Minority doctors, as the title of their report announced, were "Missing Persons."

From AMHPS's birth in 1977, the dearth of minority physician had been perhaps *the* motivating force behind the association's efforts. While the reasons for the flattening numbers in 2004 were outside the immediate influence of the AMHPS schools, the problem itself was in the association's wheelhouse. AMHPS had established a leadership role on this subject. The numbers of minority practitioners and the diversity of the health workforce was a focus of the Office, now the Center, for Minority Health and Health Disparities. But now it seemed that all the legislation that had been put in place was not playing as significant a role as had been hoped. The schools themselves had been substantially strengthened, but the problem itself had not only not disappeared; it was now worsening.

The deadly phenomenon of disparate health care had been another prime motivator for AMHPS, and a key issue for the Center for Minority Health and Health Disparities. In 1989 research into this question had been essentially nonexistent. Since then, through research grants and research endowment funds and relentless effort by both John Ruffin and AMHPS lobbyists and leaders, research into the causes and potential for amelioration had ramped up. There were more minority medical scientists, better minority research infrastructure, and increasing acceptance of the problem's legitimacy and scope.

But for all that, in the middle of the new millennium's first decade, disparate health conditions, with the consequential high rate of Black sickness and death, seemed as operative as ever. Equally distressing, despite the improved environment for research into disparities, it appeared that minority medical scientists were having a harder time accessing NIH research funds than their white peers. A study by University of Kansas professor Donna Ginther and others showed that, after controlling for educational background, experience, training, and other relevant factors, "black applicants remain 10 percentage point less likely than whites to be awarded NIH research funding."[11] Many of the Black research applicants the study looked at came from the AMHPS schools, and some came from other institutions. There seemed no ready explanation for this other than bias. "An obvious evidence of discrimination," Louis Sullivan thought.[12] "The information wasn't lost on me," said Dale Dirks. "It was very frustrating."[13]

AMHPS had a record of thinking creatively about the problems it encountered and vigorously pursuing legislation to address them. Here, then, were two challenges to AMHPS's primary objectives: increasing the numbers of minority doctors and improving the research environment for minority scientists. What strategies might be effective to address this emerging reality?

In 2007 AMHPS was thirty-years old. For most of that time Dale Dirks had been the association's chief lobbyist. He still was. But leadership at the AMHPS schools was going through a generational change, and the times themselves were very different from what they had been when the association first got started. In the wake of the civil rights movement, the 1970s had been a more militant era, and that energy hadn't bypassed the Black health professions schools. In the 1990s the successes of the Clinton administrations had brought a calmer atmosphere to Black and white relations, if not to the political arena. Pulitzer Prize winner and Nobel laureate Toni Morrison had even called Bill Clinton "the first Black president."

The AMHPS schools themselves had changed too. In the 1970s each one of the association's founding institutions had, in one way or another, been poised on a financial precipice. They were still far from robust financially. But the AMHPS-driven legislation had brought in significant amounts of federal money; it had given them all some room to breathe.

Passing time had brought with it a new environment, and also new leadership. Almost all the founders had now passed the torch to new presidents and new deans. Of the four presidents who had presented the association's manifesto to Margaret Heckler, none were still in office. Walter Bowie, Alfred Haynes, and Sullivan had retired. David Satcher had left the academic world to become surgeon general and assistant HHS secretary, then CDC director. After their tenure at AMHPS, Ronny Lancaster, John Maupin, and Barbara Hayes at Texas Southern School of Pharmacy (Maupin's successor as AMHPS chairperson) had carried on the tradition of strong advocacy. But the newer principals were less engaged, and the association's energy suffered accordingly.

It wasn't that the new institutional leaders were less capable, but their priorities as presidents and deans had shifted away from the existential necessities their predecessors had faced. They had the same huge responsibilities for managing their institutions, but they were a little more comfortable from a financial standpoint. They were the beneficiaries of the funding programs their predecessors had succeeded in putting in place: research infrastructure, loan repayments, training programs, endowments, tuition scholarships, centers of excellence. Overall, their federal funding portfolios were performing well, which gave them the space to concentrate on their more challenging budget categories and to attend to the administrative and leadership demands their institutions required of them every day.

Among the new institutional leaders who had not been around during the vast legislative efforts of their predecessors, a sense began to seep in that these federal programs feeding their bottom lines were more or less entitlements, that they would just continue automatically. These leaders had not had the experience of creating new concepts, drafting legislation, hustling for support, fighting for appropriations. They did not have the hard-earned legislative sophistication. They didn't bear the battle scars their predecessors did.

In those circumstances, AMHPS had become less of a priority than it had been. In its earlier years, school presidents and deans had come to AMHPS board meetings; now second- or third-level administrators attended, people who weren't empowered to make decisions themselves but had to refer them up the line. The hard work of lobbying for annual appropriations hadn't diminished, but that was largely in the hands of Dirks and his colleagues. The creativity that generated new initiatives was largely missing. There was still plenty of support among members of Congress, but no one was filling the shoes of the great driver of minority health legislation, Lou Stokes. As a result, AMHPS was just not in the arena in the same way it had been. And one consequence was that the disturbing issues reported later by the Ginther study on research awards and race and by the Sullivan commission's report on "missing persons" did not rouse an AMHPS response, as it might well have only a few years earlier.

~

One large goal, though, had stayed in the minds of a core group of AMHPS veterans, more or less since the National Center Act passed in 2000. While the Center did have grant-making powers and a reasonable initial budget, it's reach was still limited relative to other NIH centers and institutes. It wasn't long before Dirks, Lancaster, Satcher, Sullivan, Maupin, and Wayne Riley (Meharry's then president) began thinking about how they might elevate the National Center into a National Institute. NIH institutes had the highest level of prestige and wielded the largest budgets. An "institute" designation would give greater emphasis to the significance of health care disparities. A larger budget would enable additional studies and efforts to ameliorate the health burdens of minority communities.

Elevating the center to an institute would require the same kind of legislative act that had raised the office to a center. While there was a good deal of talk about what might be done, the veteran leaders assumed that such an objective was more aspirational than feasible. It was hard to see when the opportunity might arise or what circumstances might give weight to the immense effort that would be required in Congress. Even the fact that there was now an African American president—Barack Obama was elected in 2008—didn't really improve the prospects. In fact, AMHPS had submitted a proposal to the Obama transition team arguing the case for training more minority health care professionals and increasing funding for historically Black graduate institutions, research infrastructure, and research endowments—in essence including AMHPS programs among the ideas the Obama administration was incubating regarding health care reform. But in the press of transition business, the proposal had gained zero traction. The incoming administration had its own thoughts about health care.

Obama had identified health care reform as a key priority, and not long after the administration settled in, the new president's health team began piecing together the reform plan that eventually became the Affordable Care Act (ACA). The act, as it developed, was massive, and the negotiations over it were protracted and increasingly heated. Although the ACA's initial concepts derived largely from Heritage Foundation ideas and Massachusetts Republican governor Mitt Romney's state health plan, Republican opposition was fierce, centering on the insurance aspects of the bill.

In the midst of this monumental congressional dustup, Dirks, Lancaster, Sullivan, and their colleagues saw an opportunity.

Under ordinary circumstances, raising the center to an institute would have taken its own act—a distant prospect. But here in front of them was a giant bill covering dozens of health issues and attracting many amendments; moreover, the fight over its central provisions was sucking all the air out of the political atmosphere. Perhaps, they thought, a simple, brief amendment to the bill would attract little attention. The circumstances seemed promising.

As AMHPS started drafting an amendment that would change the National Center of Minority Health and Health Disparities into a national institute, Sullivan, Dirks, Ruffin, Lancaster, Drew president Susan Kelly, and Meharry president Wayne Riley went to see Francis Collins, the newly appointed director of NIH.

Collins was a distinguished research scientist who had headed the National Human Genome Research Institute prior to being named NIH director. Harold Varmus, the earlier NIH director, was now in Collins's place as director of the Genome Research Institute. Like Varmus, Collins was committed to NIH's rigorous peer review mechanism for determining funding priorities. And like Varmus, Collins was not a fan of the social science orientation of a good deal of health disparities research. Varmus—Sullivan, Satcher, and the others remembered it vividly—had only bowed to their arguments for the Center after a series of confrontational meetings. They also remembered that had Varmus not changed his mind and come out in favor, the Clinton administration would not have supported the National Center bill either, which would have spelled the end of the venture.

Sullivan opened the discussion, telling Collins how pleased he and the others were that the Center had developed as it had. At the same time, he said, "we believe it still doesn't have the level of support it should have. We think it's time that it should become an institute. That would give it additional prestige and a larger budget to do the essential work it's doing."

Collins was not overwhelmed by the argument. "Well," he said, "that really wouldn't have much meaning. As you know, there's no legislative authority that an institute has that's any different from what a center has. It's got a budget, grant making authority. It's got programs. I don't see what the need is to elevate it to an institute. There's really no essential difference between the two."

"In that case," said Sullivan, "if they really are functionally and administratively the same, that's all the more reason it should be an institute. If there's no difference, why not call it an institute and enable it do its work more effectively?"

"Well, said Collins, "let me think about it."[14]

Sullivan and the others never did get a firm commitment from Collins that he would support the change. They saw that as a lingering lack of NIH enthusiasm for the work the National Center was doing. On the other hand, he had not rejected the idea. And as the movement toward a vote on the Senate floor gathered momentum, Collins decided not to oppose the amendment. He probably thought, Sullivan reflected later, that there was no point in coming out in opposition. It wasn't an issue of principle for him. Besides, the country had a new Black president. There was nothing to be gained in risking a negative reaction from that quarter.

The amendment that Dirks and his colleague Lodriguez Murray drafted was a model of simplicity and brevity. Every place where the overall health law mentioned the National Center for Minority Health and Health Disparities, the amendment substituted "Institute" for "Center." (Each HHS agency also had its administratively established minority health office. The amendment wrote each of them into law so that they couldn't be arbitrarily eliminated.)

With the amendment written, Dirks approached Maryland's Senator Ben Cardin, who had previously demonstrated support for minority health care matters. Two days later Cardin's staff got back to him. The senator agreed to sponsor the amendment. Shortly afterward the Affordable Care Act came to the Senate floor for debate, and Cardin offered the amendment. There was essentially no discussion; and when the ACA passed, the National Center for Minority Health and Health Disparities took its place as one of NIH's twenty national institutes.

CHAPTER 11

A Common Mission

The elevation of NIH's National Center on Minority Health and Health Disparities to an institute was a major step in terms of budget and, equally significant, in terms of gaining recognition for the importance of the new institute's central mission. Minority health and health disparities were now NIH key issues and had been formally declared as such as prominently as possible. This happened in 2010, a quarter century after Margaret Heckler issued her report on the perilous discrepancies between minority and white morbidity and mortality. Earlier in his directorship, John Ruffin had had difficulty convincing people that health disparities were real, not some imagined fiction. There was still an enduring strain of resistance at NIH to the new institute's mission, but outright skepticism about the reality and depth of the problem was disappearing. Paula Braveman, a member of Ruffin's advisory council, saw that health disparities issues had become more mainstream. "Most physicians have at least heard of the term," she said. "[They] have some awareness of the magnitude and pervasiveness of the health disparities between members of minority groups and white Americans."[1]

Bringing that recognition into the medical mainstream was largely an AMHPS accomplishment. AMHPS had conceived and fostered the National Center Act. Then AMHPS had found a way to elevate the center into an institute as part of the Affordable Care Act; Dale Dirks and his associates had drafted the amendment and found a sponsor. The long struggle to bring health disparities from invisibility into the light was gaining ground, at least in the medical and medical science community. But, after the programs established by the National Center Act in 2000—endowments, loan repayment, centers of excellence—were in place, no meaningful new legislation had come out of the AMHPS leadership. The yearly lobbying effort to keep the already-established programs funded was ongoing, but the legislative creativity that had always distinguished AMHPS had, to all intents and purposes, played itself out.

Nowhere was this more evident than in the response to the Donna Ginther journal article, "Race, Ethnicity, and NIH Research Awards," which found that minority investigators were far less likely to receive NIH grants than were their white peers. This was a deeply disturbing finding, but from AMHPS there was no response. By contrast, a small organization composed of senior African American professors in academic medicine (the Association for Academic Minority Physicians, AAMP), founded by University of Maryland School of Medicine dean Donald Wilson, applied to NIH for a grant to set up mentoring programs for minority researchers. The response wasn't what they hoped for, but NIH did fund a five-year, so called P-50 research program grant based at Boston College (AAMP was a subrecipient) that did give rise to a national network of mentors.

There was a time, not that many years before the Ginther study, when AMHPS leaders would have shaped a legislative proposal and begun gathering congressional support. "We would have jumped right on that," said former AMHPS president Ronny Lancaster.[2] By contrast, the 1999 report by a committee led by Alfred Haynes on the miniscule number of National Cancer Institute dollars spent on minority disease had triggered congressional hearings and had sparked the drive to elevate the Office of Research on Minority Health into a center. Now, when it was clear that minority researchers were being sidetracked by NIH in their quest for funding, AMHPS was silent.

That nothing was forthcoming now was telling. Nurturing young minority researchers had been a leading AMHPS objective. Loan repayment programs had helped minority schools attract young faculty; the Research Centers in Minority Institutions (RCMI) Act had given AMHPS schools the wherewithal to build advanced research facilities and bring in "magnet" scientists together with their junior associates and trainees. The RCMI Act had established high-level research collaborations among the minority schools. The centers of excellence programs had given AMHPS and other minority-serving schools key roles in research that furthered the health of minorities. At the heart of the National Center Act, the research endowment program not only made grants available, but built up permanent research funding. AMHPS schools had always seen the nurturing of Black investigators as a central issue, and the association had historically responded to the need by generating legislation and doing the hard work of getting it through committees and floor votes and signed into law. But now the energy for that had seemingly dissipated.

Since its first engagement with the legislative process in the 1980s, the AMHPS schools had considered medical science, and especially young medical science investigators, a priority. But they had also paid special attention to the beginning of the pipeline—the young people who were prime candidates for careers. The dearth of Black researchers was a stark reality going back as far as anyone cared to look. But as AMHPS ramped up its agenda in the mid-1980s, the leaders decided that something needed to be done to attract young minds to the excitement, satisfactions, and importance of biomedical research. They saw such an endeavor as a long-term effort, one that would bear fruit in the numbers and quality of applicants to their schools.

Walter Sullivan, Louis Sullivan's older brother, led the AMHPS endeavor, which became known as the Symposium on Career Opportunities in Biomedical and Public Health Sciences. Walter Sullivan was a PhD chemist who had done his graduate work at Ohio State University and had been a professor, department chair, and dean at several Southern universities. In 1985 he was vice president for operations and planning at Morehouse School of Medicine. Sullivan envisioned a program that would introduce large numbers of minority young people to the health sciences by exposing them to highly accomplished Black and Latino figures who could talk about their work and show them that a path was open to careers in these fields.

The biomedical symposia, as Walter Sullivan and his AMHPS colleagues conceived them, would invite promising minority students to an all-expense-paid extended weekend in one of the cities where an AMHPS school was located. Eleventh- and twelfth-grade high school students and first- and second-year college students would be eligible—young people thinking about their futures, many who had never given any consideration to careers as scientists, largely because they had never seen or heard that Black people were welcomed in science professions. At these symposia students would hear talks by distinguished Black and Latino medical scientists and attend seminars and workshops run by minority individuals who were making careers for themselves in academic medicine. The students would see, hear, and talk to "people who looked like them," as Sullivan put it, doing exciting things with their lives in fields few of the student attendees had ever dreamed might be available to them. "I wanted to captivate them," Sullivan said. "I wanted to stir a fever in them."[3]

These gatherings, Walter Sullivan and his colleagues hoped, would help increase the trickle of Black and minority students who were able to find their way through the barriers that stood in the way of pursuing careers in health and medical science. As far as academic medicine was concerned, that was hardly even a trickle. In the mid-1970s, when Morehouse School of Medicine was founded, there were scarcely more than a dozen African Americans in American academic medicine outside the few Black health professions schools. Ten years later, when Walter Sullivan launched the biomedical symposia, the numbers were better but still meager.

In 1988 Sullivan approached NIH for funding and received a grant from the National Institute of General Medical Sciences that enabled him to launch his first symposium in Nashville, Tennessee, home to Meharry Medical College. Three hundred or so students attended. Walter Bowie was one of two keynote speakers; the other was Louis Sullivan, Walter's brother. The two AMHPS's founders had themselves been prominent medical scientists before taking on their current roles—Bowie as dean at Tuskegee's veterinary school, Sullivan as president at Morehouse.

With the success of the first gathering, the following year Walter Sullivan applied for a larger grant. The second event was held in Los Angeles, home to Charles Drew University of Medicine and Science. A thousand students attended. In the following years, attendance grew to fifteen hundred, and then two thousand and more. The excitement among the student attendees was palpable. In consecutive years the country's two leading neurosurgeons spoke, Keith Black from Cedars-Sinai Medical Center in Los Angeles and Ben Carson from Johns Hopkins, both African Americans. Another year the students heard from Dr. Mae Jemison, the first African American female NASA astronaut, and another year from PhD veterinarian (and Miss America) Debbye Turner.

The events generated excitement among the schools' faculties and administrators as well, and the symposia became featured events on the schools' calendars. NIH grants increased to support the growth in attendance, transportation costs, first class hotel stays, and honoraria for speakers and workshop leaders (which were usually declined). From early on, the NIH money was supplemented by donations from companies like Exxon, Dow Corning, and Amgen, whose scientists also took part.

While AMHPS regarded these programs as potentially important contributors to their member schools and to Black medicine and health in general, the biomedical symposia also had an emotional effect on the schools' deans, presidents, and senior leadership. Most members of this group were born and raised in the South in the 1920s and '30s when there had been almost no possibility for them to undertake graduate or professional training in their home region, except at HBCUs (Historically Black Colleges and Universities). Mainstream Southern schools' doors were shut tight against Black enrollment. As a result, many had pursued their advanced studies in the North. But Northern schools themselves ordinarily admitted few Blacks, which meant they often found themselves the sole African American among their classmates. They frequently had no Black peers in their entire schools; most had never in their lives encountered a Black professor.

When Walter Sullivan had done his doctoral work in chemistry at Ohio State, he was the single Black chemistry graduate student. His brother Louis had been the only African American in his class at Boston University School of Medicine. When David Satcher entered the MD/PhD program at Case Western University in Cleveland, he had no Black classmates, nor did Norman Francis, who integrated Louisiana's Loyola University. When Louis Sullivan was an intern at Cornell's New York Hospital, one day he saw another young African American wearing a white coat and a stethoscope across a ward. The two men eyed each other quizzically and said at the same time, "What are you doing here?" (The other trainee was Alvin Poussaint, who later became an internationally known psychiatrist and associate dean at Harvard Medical School.) For individuals who had gone through the isolation of those experiences, seeing thousands of Black young people meeting with accomplished Black health professionals was deeply moving.

AMPHS was now working both ends of the field, with the biomedical symposia for high schoolers and undergraduates on one end and its push for research funding and the means to attract young investigators on the other. They were inspiring young potential scientists and enlarging opportunities for graduate scientists. Both endeavors traced their origins back to the late 1980s. But by 2005 AMHPS's efforts in both fields had withered. Walter Sullivan ran the biomedical symposia until 2002, when Carol Lewis, formerly on the CDC staff, took over. When several years later Lewis became ill, the program dwindled quickly. The enthusiasm of the participants hadn't flagged, but the energy necessary to sustain the symposia had simply given out. The two thousand student attendees had decreased to one hundred, and by 2006 the biomedical symposia were discontinued. Nor by then was AMHPS developing new legislation to advance African

American researchers. The result was that both ends of the field that had once been worked so vigorously now stood neglected.

~

Shutting down the biomedical symposia was a token of the fall-off in creativity and energy. It was also the elimination of a bond that helped keep the coalition of schools together. AMHPS's successes had been contingent on an understanding—and a conviction—that all the minority health professions schools, in medicine, dentistry, pharmacy, and veterinary medicine were engaged in essentially the same fight for the recognition of Black health needs and the creation of a Black health force that could better serve the minority population and could also find its place in the national endeavor to better the health of the American people generally. To the AMHPS founders it had been obvious that these objectives could be pursued more effectively together than separately. That belief had been borne out. But with the well of creativity drying up, the power of coalition action began to seem less relevant—except in the business of lobbying to fund already-existing programs, which in the extreme contentiousness that increasingly characterized the political world was itself becoming a far more laborious process.

Currently the decline in AMHPS's effectiveness has continued. "The major challenge," according to Rueben Warren, director of the National Center for Bioethics in Research and Health Care at Tuskegee University, "is the sense of separation that was created in the latter years because the new leadership that came in did not understand the essential nature of functioning as one unit. They saw them themselves, in my view, as individual institutions as opposed to the collective. Their sense of connectedness was lost."[4]

At the same time, the driving issues that had propelled AMHPS into existence in 1977 were still afflicting communities of color in 2021, more than forty years later. AMHPS's founding white paper had identified the two fundamental problems that had struck the association's founders with such force. "Historically," Louis Sullivan had written in the preface to *Blacks and the Health Professions in the '80s: A National Crisis and a Time for Action*, "there has been, and there continues to be, a severe shortage of black health professionals in the United States." "Blacks," he wrote, "have more illness and a significantly shorter life expectancy than do whites in the United States." In 2022 (as this book goes to press), the African American community still suffers from an ongoing shortage of Black health professionals, a greater burden of disease, and shorter life spans than their white fellow citizens. The crisis has not disappeared, nor has the need for action.

The 1970s were a time defined by signature events in the life of the nation. Civil rights laws had been passed prohibiting racial discrimination in employment, public accommodation, housing, and voting. Martin Luther King Jr.'s assassination had sent shock waves through the country and had raised the consciousnesses of large numbers of Americans and American institutions. Laws were being implemented; customs and habits of mind were changing. The radical departures of the mid-1960s had begun to settle in as norms. Social justice had thrust itself forward as a theme, in the foreground for some and at least in the background ambience for many others. The business of racial equality as a principle in everyday life informed the debate over what it meant to be an American as it never previously had. It was in these circumstances that the AMHPS schools had mounted their case for more minority health professionals and an assault on the disparities that afflicted Black health and shortened Black lives. The time was right. In Congress the message resonated on both sides of the aisle.

In 2020 another defining period had arrived. Its social manifestation was called Black Lives Matter, but the awareness the name signified had been gathering momentum for a number of years with the deaths of unarmed African Americans at the hands of police. Police use of deadly force was, of course, part of the world of law enforcement, but some of the fatal encounters highlighted on social media and cell phone videos showed blatantly unwarranted police killings. The emotional buildup engendered by these incidents affected both Blacks and whites.

In August, 2020, already-heightened anger and distress exploded into massive demonstrations with the police murder of George Floyd, choked to death on a Minneapolis street and shown on national television. Black Lives Matter became a rallying cry nationally, on the streets, in the media, on signs and placards in windows and on lawns. In the highly politicized climate of the Donald Trump administration, it was impossible to tell how deeply or widely Black Lives Matter sentiments actually affected the general public, but there was no doubt that the issue of racial derogation and injustice was illuminated as it had not been in the half century since King's death.

The heightened attention given to racism and its pervasive impact on society generated a surge in media inquiries into slavery and the lasting damage that has been slavery's legacy. In addition, largely forgotten nineteenth- and early twentieth-century massacres of Blacks became national news, including prominently the 1921 destruction of Tulsa's prosperous Black district of Greenwood, which killed three hundred people and eradicated the Black economy there.

By 2020 this confluence of emotionally charged current events and past racist enormities had amplified national thinking about the pressures that affect the lives and well-being of African Americans. Then the COVID-19 pandemic revealed an even larger picture of Black inequality, measured in the numbers of those the virus had sickened and killed. The disproportionate share of suffering borne by the minority populations brought the problem of health disparities into the light of public knowledge as it simply never had been before. As of October 2020, the number of Black Americans who had died of COVID-19 was 43,844, an actual mortality rate twice that of white Americans, and an age-adjusted mortality rate 3.2 times higher than that of white Americans.[5]

~

The stark picture drawn by the pandemic's impact crystallized the matter of health disparities and what they meant in real life. In 2005 David Satcher and colleagues had published a report on the African American death rate compared to the white death rate. The study was published in *Health Affairs*, a health policy research journal.[6] Now data on Black deaths were no longer embedded in a scholarly journal, they were broadcast to the public. Black Lives Matter was the slogan of a social movement, but "Black lives matter" had been the central theme of AMHPS from its beginning.

In 2020, the question was, did the awareness of disease and death generated by the pandemic create the circumstances that would reinvigorate AMHPS and renew the association's decades-long campaign for equity in health? Or, had AMHPS served its purpose as a leader on this subject and was now simply a formal structure rather than a force for action?

For John Ruffin, the long-time former director of the National Institute on Minority Health and Health Disparities, the urgency was manifest.

> The pandemic has peeled back attention to what Lou Sullivan and others have been talking about for years and years and years. We're talking now about exactly the same thing, exactly the same issues. We can't wait on other people to solve this for us. We need to create the infrastructure and have some place where we can speak up. We have got to do this ourselves. We can't wait on a [former acting NIH

director] Ruth Kirschstein who supported us or a Harold Varmus, with whom we had both disagreements and agreements. We have to do this ourselves. Right now. A lot of those people that we helped produce from the Centers of Excellence and from people that we trained with the funds from the endowment and the loan repayments, they've got to come forward and say, we need to do this. We need to be involved.[7]

When Ruffin speaks of the need for an "infrastructure" and "some place where we can speak up," it's impossible not to think that AMHPS has historically provided exactly that infrastructure and platform. Others who have played leading roles in AMHPS and in minority health care generally have similar thoughts about the urgency of the moment. They make the point that the reality of health inequities has never resonated in the same way prior to this period and that AMHPS has unique strengths to bring to this and other issues of minority health.

～

The concept of AMHPS and its inherent strength still features largely in the minds of the older generation of leaders—Satcher, Sullivan, Warren, Lancaster, John Maupin. These are people who have dealt with the same or similar problems for many years and who built a robust organization to address them. AMHPS, the organization they built, had historic significance in terms of the evolution of Black health professionals and health care. The organization still carries great symbolic weight for this older generation, embodying as it does the concept of African American connectedness, mutual aid, and the power that unity brings to political, cultural, and legislative action.

If there is a consensus about the prerequisite for a renewal of AMHPS as a catalyst in minority health, it is that the member institutions need to revive their commitment to united action rather than to their individual interests. That's not any easy proposition. The association that came together in 1977 was composed of schools driven by financial need. Funding, they saw then, could be accessed more successfully as members of a coalition rather than as individual institutions. That existential driver no longer obtains. The other side of it is that the schools now have at their disposal the hard-earned knowledge of how to work together for mutual benefit, even if that knowledge has been little utilized in recent years.

The past furnishes the AMHPS institutions with possibilities for renewing the cross-institutional ties that once bound them, in essence, reintegrating themselves. The biomedical symposia, for example, were hugely successful and energized the sense of collective identity. One of the problems in sustaining them was that they were funded by NIH grants, which needed to be renewed yearly, and by corporate donations, which needed to be sought out and administered.

The endeavor was labor-intensive, and dependence on soft money strained the association's capabilities. But could a program, perhaps one that included students from socially, educationally, and economically disadvantaged white communities, be funded by congressional action? Rueben Warren at Tuskegee's Center for Bioethics in Research and Health Care believes an endeavor of that sort might well be "legislatively fundable." Robert Byrd would certainly have approved. Today's legislators from Appalachia might also. AMHPS is a small organization that has always punched above its weight, primarily by mustering congressional support from cities and states where minority health professions schools are located. Expanding the base of students would also expand AMHPS's political reach.

Another mutual endeavor among AMHPS member schools might be the *Journal of Health Care for the Poor and Underserved.*

Satcher founded this journal when he was president of Meharry. When John Maupin succeeded Satcher, he revamped the journal and arranged for the Johns Hopkins University Press to assume publication. If the AMHPS schools were to adopt the journal as their official publication, it would provide a venue for discussion of the goals and interests of the member schools, a platform for commentary on minority health issues and needed congressional action, and a showcase for studies and scholarship coming out of the AMHPS institutions. It would give AMHPS a voice that could carry significant weight. In the Project Muse database of 709 refereed journals in all areas of arts and sciences, the *Journal of Health Care for the Poor and Underserved* is number four in terms of readership. So AMHPS would not only have a unified voice, it would have a vastly amplified voice.

AMHPS's original lead issues were the shortage of Black health professionals and the disparities in health and health care. Those issues drove the AMHPS agenda and led directly to legislation strengthening the schools and to the creation of an NIH office (then center, then institute) established to investigate minority health and disparities. Those issues are no less grave today, but AMHPS is not playing a lead role, or perhaps any role, in addressing them. Investigators from the individual institutions apply for grants, but grant proposals from a Meharry or Xavier have a hard time competing against proposals from Harvard or Johns Hopkins. The minority schools simply do not match up in resources or standing. The frustration is evident when a large proposal from Xavier University College of Pharmacy, for example, loses out to one from Harvard or Hopkins, despite Xavier's intimate connection with and understanding of the minority community.

"We can't wait on other people to solve this for us," says Ruffin. "We have to do this ourselves."[8] The frustration evident in Ruffin's comment is shared by others; the problem is finding a solution. The AMHPS schools have a history of acting together when individual resources are insufficient. In 1986, for example, RCMI administrator Sidney McNairy established a series of collaborative centers for AMHPS schools that enabled sophisticated gene sequencing studies. Pooling resources for large studies on health disparities might well give research proposals the additional heft they need to succeed in NIH's rigorous review process. Collaborative work by definition would augment the sense of connection among the schools.

The same may be true regarding AMHPS's other original lead issue: the dearth of minority health professionals. In some ways that situation has changed during AMHPS's lifetime. By the early 1970s the civil rights laws with their equal access mandates were kicking in, Northern medical school doors had opened, and even schools in the South were bowing to the inevitable and integrating themselves. In the 1970s and 1980s African American enrollment in medical schools saw regular increases. But at the end of the 1980s the numbers began to plateau; as a percentage of total medical school enrollment, they have not increased since then. Today (2020) approximately 7.5 percent of medical school enrollees are Black, while Blacks account for almost 13 percent of the US population. Almost all of the increase in Black medical school enrollees is an increase in the number of Black female students. In terms of numbers, Black males lag badly. This is an issue in AMHPS's wheelhouse. It is a question whether the AMHPS schools should not be addressing this issue through a combined effort to understand why it's happening and to devise nationally applicable strategies to solve it.

∼

While it is possible to identify both discrete programs, like the biomedical symposia, and broad scope issues, such as health disparities and the shortage of minority health professionals, the grand theme that ties all the minority schools together can perhaps best be described as a "social mission." If the AMHPS schools have a common vision, it is that from their beginnings, each has in one way or another been driven by the desire to provide care for a Black community in severe need. The founding stories of Howard, Meharry, Tuskegee, Xavier, Morehouse, Drew, Hampton, Florida A&M, and Texas Southern all incorporate that basic theme.

In health care terms, "social mission" refers to the percentage of graduates who practice primary care and work in areas with a shortage of health professionals. "Social mission" schools further diversity among health professionals and encourage reforms tending toward social justice. (It's worth noting that the new charter of the American College of Physicians identifies social justice as one of its fundamental principles.) A study out of George Washington University School of Medicine and Health Sciences showed that by these criteria many of the most prestigious medical schools in the country rank in the bottom part of the list. The number one school for social mission was determined to be Morehouse School of Medicine. The number two school was Meharry Medical College. The number three school was Howard University College of Medicine.[9]

"If they had asked that question about the top pharmacy schools," said Tuskegee's Rueben Warren, "the answer would have been the same. It would have been the same for dental schools too." The AMHPS schools would have dominated the social mission rankings in those health fields as well. "That study verified that there is a common mission. But the common mission is sometimes lost," says Warren. "It's not articulated any more. George Washington University had to report that rather than the AMHPS schools articulating it to Congress. That would have been a strategy rather than a finding published in a medical journal. Instead, the debate in the schools' inner circles was about which one was really first, second or third—instead of 'Look what we have done together!' The conversation needs to be about the common vision. Not a Morehouse vision or a Meharry vision or a Howard vision. I'm not sure," says Warren, "that that conversation is taking place."[10]

At the same time, according to the George Washington study, NIH funding to medical schools was inversely associated with social mission scores. That is, the higher a school's social mission was ranked, the less NIH funding that school received. The study authors (the lead author was George Washington University professor of health policy and pediatrics, Fitzhugh Mullan) concluded, "Medical schools vary substantially in their contribution to the social mission of medical education. . . . These findings suggest that initiatives at the medical school level could increase the proportion of physicians who practice primary care, work in underserved areas, and are [themselves] underrepresented minorities."[11]

There is already, in 2021, a severe shortage of primary care physicians, which is worse in traditionally underserved areas. Current predictions are that by 2033, twelve years from now, the shortage will grow alarmingly. The Association of American Medical Colleges projects a shortfall of between 21,400 and 55,200 primary care physicians. Again, AMHPS has past experience that bears on this situation. Thirty-three years ago, the association conceived and carried through Congress the Excellence in Minority Health Education and Care Act, which recognized and rewarded the historic contribution of minority health professions schools to public health by training primary care health professionals to serve in areas with shortages.

The minority schools still need strengthening in this regard in order to sustain and upgrade their primary care training programs. But looking beyond their own programs, Morehouse, Meharry, and Howard are the national models for the principle of social mission in medical schools; they have long experience in incentivizing the development of primary care physicians for service among the neediest populations. The same is true of the AMHPS dental, pharmacy, and veterinary schools. Legislation that recognizes their leadership in this crucial area and provides funding for promulgating best ideas and practices would seem a natural direction for the AMHPS institutions. But, as Warren suggests, such a development would only be possible if the schools renewed their commitment to unity and combined action.

~

If it is true that because COVID-19 has conveyed such a powerful impression of disparate health and because Black Lives Matter has changed the conversation about race, we may well be at an inflection point in our conception of ourselves as a nation, just as we were in the late 1960s after the civil rights laws and the death of Martin Luther King Jr. As the 1950s and '60s are called the civil rights era, we may now be seeing the advent of the social justice era. Time will reveal if that is or is not overly optimistic. But if this is a true inflection point, then the AMHPS schools' stature as models for social justice in health care may well point toward a more active role than has been the case recently.

What might that more active role look like? Certainly there is the opportunity to expand the scope of AMHPS in terms of embracing the new realities of health care: the extension of primary care through nurses, nurse practitioners, and physicians assistants, for example, and the growing significance of community-based health centers. Expanding the reach of health care available in underserved communities is AMHPS's reason for existing. Now, more than forty years after the association's founding, that is still its reason for existing, but the realities on the ground have evolved. Can AMHPS see its role as building leadership resources to create legislation that furthers grassroots primary health care? Morehouse

School of Medicine has a National Center for Primary Care. Is that an expandable concept, for example, that might generate new capabilities and spread benefits to all the AMHPS schools?

Again, there's precedent for this in AMHPS's experience. The original Title III expansion to extend federal support from undergraduate to graduate institutions was specifically designed to assist Morehouse School of Medicine. Subsequently, other AMHPS schools were folded in, then other nonmedical HBCUs. Today eighteen institutions benefit from funding that supports training for students in many fields of professional life. The initial narrow focus broadened to include many more schools and many more disciplines.

The Research Centers in Minority Institutions (RCMI) Act is another example. Initially limited to Black graduate institutions, it expanded to include institutions that serve other minority groups, including disadvantaged white communities in largely rural states where research infrastructure is not well-developed. That was Robert Byrd's intention when he gave his support to what became a national center on not just minority health but also on health disparities. Disadvantaged white constituents who benefit from the program help preserve interest and funding support long-term. They strengthen its political appeal.

AMHPS-inspired programs have regularly expanded from a narrow focus on minority schools to an embrace of non–African American communities. That seems to have been an organic feature of their development. AMHPS leaders haven't objected to this. It might not have been part of their intention, but at the same time they have a natural affinity with other communities suffering similar health inequities. "I not only do not object to that," says Louis Sullivan, "I agree with it. I think expansion of that sort shows in graphic detail that Blacks and other minorities can contribute to programs that not only benefit them, but benefit broader society. . . . [T]hese novel contributions by a small segment of society often grow to the benefit of all."[12]

~

The idea of embracing the wider community indicates another potential path forward for AMHPS. "Social mission" is not a racial term. The National Center on Minority Health and Health Disparities, whose mission was broadened to include underserved white populations through what might be called the Robert Byrd Principle, within several years also identified women, veterans, LGBTQ individuals, and other groups as qualifying for its benefits. The partnerships AMHPS built with other organizations in the past can easily be rekindled and amplified by new partnerships with organizations representing groups that have significant common interests in health equity. With a larger community of partners, there would be more leverage for advancing policy and legislative initiatives that have the potential to bring in new resources. The time during the pandemic and post-pandemic may create important opportunities for growth.

Expansion in terms of embracing new avenues to primary care or of new partner organizations would give AMHPS greater leverage in pursuing its primary goals. But to do that, the prerequisite is leadership with creativity and vision, which will only be forthcoming if substantial incentives become obvious. The alternative is to maintain the current level of activity, which is mainly to continue lobbying for funding for existing legislation. The chosen alternative will determine how AMHPS will be assessed in the ongoing story of Black health care and its long American journey.

~

AMHPS was born as a revolutionary coalition in a time of great challenges and great opportunities. In that environment, the minority health professions schools leveraged their common strength to shore themselves up financially and to acquire the kinds of infrastructure and human resources that enhanced their status and gave them a voice in the national conversation about health and health care. They brought to that conversation concerns that are now considered fundamental but previously were little noted. They introduced, through the AMHPS-inspired Heckler Report, the concept that the federal government is responsible for the health of the country's minority peoples. They brought to the nation's attention the harsh realities of disparate care and the obligation to do something about it. They increased awareness of the lack of minority practitioners and the pressing problem of inadequate professional care in rural and inner-city America.

AMHPS brought these concerns to the attention of the country's medical and scientific establishments and to the public generally. If today we are talking about disparate care, we have AMHPS largely to thank. If we are trying to remedy the inequities suffered by the nation's minority and poor white populations, AMHPS has been at the forefront. If the social obligation of the health profession has become a subject, AMHPS's role has been consequential. If we are thinking about the value of all lives, that has been AMHPS's great theme.

These are signal accomplishments, brought about by an organization whose establishment was itself a signal accomplishment. The long and hard history of Blacks and American medicine saw the emergence of Black physicians in pre–Civil War times and the trickle of Black doctors, dentists and pharmacists growing to a small stream by the latter part of the nineteenth century. The barriers to inclusion they encountered in the mainstream of the health system they overcame by creating their own local and national associations. In so doing they asserted their legitimacy and amplified their voices. Their story traces the long march from isolation and relegation to community and empowerment. That same story of emergence, isolation, and struggle for recognition was told by the Black health institutions as well. And for the Black schools of medicine, dentistry, pharmacy, and veterinary medicine, the fragility of the individual institutions was transformed into the strength they found in unity.

That is the story (to date) of the Association of Minority Health Professions Schools, a culmination of sorts in this ongoing historical narrative. But as unique as AMHPS's existence and achievements have been, the question posed now, in the third decade of the twenty-first century, has to do not with Black medicine or health care but with the life cycle of organizations. Some organizations thrive, achieve, and then inevitably succumb to the centrifugal forces that fray their bonds and sap their vitality. Others take stock of new realities and find ways to overcome their deficiencies and recommit themselves to the work they undertook at the start.

AMHPS is today a case in point. George Floyd and the Black Lives Matter movement have created a social justice environment that is like nothing since the civil rights era and the aftermath of Martin Luther King Jr.'s murder. The health care dimension of that shift in national thinking has been blown into prominence by the blatant disparities revealed by the COVID-19 pandemic. To address the deadly shortfalls in minority care, Black and other minority physicians and organizations have mobilized their efforts. But there is no single group in the country that wields the same credibility in the Black community as do the minority health professions schools. Nor is there a group more dedicated to ameliorating the special health problems of the Black community, most particularly when these institutions act together as a single unit. And *that* is their challenge going forward.

Afterword

The Association of Minority Health Professions Schools (AMHPS) was organized during a unique period of social and political change in the United States, in the second half of the twentieth century. It was during this time that racial segregation in public schools was declared unconstitutional by the US Supreme Court, the Marshall Plan was organized by the US government to rebuild war ravaged Europe, the GI Bill was created to assist our military personnel with their return to civilian life, the Interstate Highway System was constructed to facilitate the efficient movement of people and goods around the country, and the civil rights movement, led by Martin Luther King Jr. and others, reached its pinnacle. In the decades after World War II, the United States changed in ways that would have challenged the imaginations of the country's citizens when the war began.

In health care too the nation was seeing major changes. With population growth and the rising demand for medical services, in the1950s the country was facing a dramatic future shortage of physicians. In response to this projected physician shortage, the federal government began to promote the expansion of medical education. Funds were provided for student scholarships and loans, construction of medical school facilities, support of faculty, curriculum innovations, and biomedical research. These activities resulted in doubling the number of physicians graduating annually from US medical schools, from 8,000 in 1950 to more than 16,000 in 1981. The number of US medical schools increased from 80 in 1950 to 127 by 1981. Among the 47 new medical schools were two predominantly African American schools: Morehouse School of Medicine in Atlanta (charter class admitted in 1978) and the Charles R. Drew Postgraduate Medical School in Los Angeles (charter class admitted in 1981). Among the 80 existing schools were two predominately African American medical schools: Howard in Washington, DC, and Meharry in Nashville, Tennessee, which had been founded in the nineteenth century, along with more than 150 Black colleges (Historically Black Colleges and Universities, HBCUs) founded to educate the newly freed slaves.

In 1977, the nation's predominantly African American health professions schools formed the Association of Minority Health Professions Schools (AMHPS) to work in a coordinated way to secure specific programs and funding from the US government and other sources. Like HBCUs, predominantly African American health professions schools had chronically received less financial support from public and private sources than had white health professions schools.

The membership of AMHPS grew from four institutions in 1977 (Morehouse School of Medicine, Meharry Medical College, Tuskegee School of Veterinary Medicine, and Xavier University College of Pharmacy) to twelve institutions by 1995, comprising all of the nation's predominantly African American schools of medicine, dentistry, veterinary medicine, and pharmacy.

This level of institutional collaboration made it possible to promote new programs and secure funding for the schools to increase their faculties, students, facilities, scholarships, student loans, and research programs. In addition, the activities of AMHPS over a period of twenty years (1990–2010) led to the creation of the National Institute on Minority Health and Health Disparities (NIMHD) at NIH. In 2020 NIMHD celebrated its tenth anniversary and is supporting research on the etiology of disparities in health status and in access to health care for the nation's minority and poor populations.

AMHPS has been successful working with advocates and supporters in the US Congress (members of the Congressional Black Caucus, the chairs and ranking members of committees on health, appropriations, agriculture, etc.). AMHPS also formed liaisons with private health advocacy organizations such as Research!America, the American Lung Association, the American Cancer Society, and others. AMHPS was an active supporter of the successful effort led by Research!America to double the annual federal appropriation for the National Institutes of Health from 1999 to 2003.

AMHPS has demonstrated the power of collaboration among institutions to achieve a common purpose. The array of new or expanded initiatives is impressive, and many of them have benefited other health programs in urban and rural areas. Included among these are the Research Centers in Minority Institutions (RCMI) program, the graduate sciences education programs of the Higher Education Act, the Research Mentoring program of NIH, and others. Key to these successes has been the active participation of the AMHPS leaders—the presidents and deans—of the health professions schools. These influential leaders have engaged in meetings at the White House, interacted with members of Congress, and attended AMHPS strategy sessions.

In all of its activities, AMHPS has been able to "punch above its weight" because of the dedication and participation of its institutional leaders and its partnership with other advocacy organizations, both Democratic and Republican. AMHPS has had excellent relations and communications with both Democratic and Republican administrations.

AMHPS has succeeded because of its vision and its commitment to a better America, and to serving all Americans, while giving special focus to minorities and the poor in our society. This has been its animating vision.

⁓

As AMHPS considers the future, it needs to take stock of the circumstances that confront the minority and poor population now and going forward, and it needs to determine how to respond to those circumstances. In the late fall of 2020, as we were writing this book, America was facing a dark winter of surging COVID-19 deaths, even as the country looked to the vaccines that eventually helped mitigate the pandemic.

It was already well-established that the virus had stricken the minority communities with special severity. When the minority health professions schools look at a health crisis like the COVID-19 pandemic, they must ask, What, if anything, can we do to counter this? Can we mobilize ourselves in some fashion to diminish our community's vulnerability? If the minority health professions schools can answer that, it may provide a new perspective on their traditional response to health disparities in general.

It is a common assumption that Black distrust of the medical establishment—growing out of a history of exclusion, prejudice, and, not least, medical experimentation on Blacks such as the Tuskegee syphilis study—is responsible for the reluctance to take vaccines promoted by today's medical establishment. If distrust is a primary motivator, then the question is: How can we break through that distrust?

In this regard the minority health schools wield great untapped power. Their teaching, their research, and their clinical work are no different in quality from the commonly accepted standards. Their curricula, their patient care, their research protocols are the same as the curricula, patient care, and protocols at predominantly white, mainstream medical schools. The medical education at Morehouse School of Medicine is very similar to that at Harvard Medical School. But the minority schools are distinct from the mainstream schools in that they are organic to the minority community. That is, they are ideally placed to break through the distrust of the minority community toward the health establishment. One might ask, for example, would a task force on vaccination organized from the minority health professions schools be effective at communicating the importance of vaccination to the minority community? Would it be persuasive in that regard? The answer is yes, it would for most minority individuals.

Likewise, could minority schools organize cross-institutional task forces to address some of the other salient problems of African American health? Infant mortality, for example, which is 2.3 times higher for Black babies as for white babies. The point here would be to pool resources, not just to understand the problem but to act on the problem, for example, to push for legislation to fund pilot programs, and to actively participate in those pilot programs in the cities that are home to the predominantly Black health schools and their affiliated hospitals. Here again, the minority schools would likely have unique outreach credibility in the affected minority community.

The same model could as easily apply to other areas of health where African Americans suffer significant disparities compared to whites, in breast cancer, for example, or prostate cancer or hypertension. AMHPS as an association has historically identified problems, figured out ways of confronting them, and then originated and pushed legislation to fund programs addressing these problems. The thrust of AMHPS's efforts has been to bring health disparities from invisibility to visibility, then to find ways to strengthen the institutions in terms of their human, infrastructure, and research resources. However, the AMHPS schools have not traditionally mobilized efforts across their institutions to focus on specific problems nor have they mobilized themselves across their institutions to undertake frontline, on-the-ground action. Yet here is where their credibility lies and their great, untapped strength. The challenge, then, is for the institutions AMHPS represents to recognize and embrace the power that their combined voice has in the African American community and to develop effective strategies for using that voice to address the health problems that afflict African Americans in particular.

The minority health professions institutions' great potential derives from the community they are part of. History has shown that the advances made by the predominantly African American schools have regularly extended their benefits to other minorities and to other impoverished, underserved populations. In the course of extending this protective umbrella, AMHPS has acted as a moral compass, helping influence the direction of mainstream schools and the medical establishment generally. In this way AMHPS has made its contribution to the progressive realization of the American creed of equality and the attainment of what the Declaration so memorably, and indelibly, described as the inalienable rights of all the nation's citizens.

But the realities that drove the minority health professions schools when they first banded together have evolved over the years. The leadership of the AMHPS schools has changed too. The founding generation has given way to different leaders in an ongoing changing of the guard over almost forty-five years. New leaders have confronted different institutional challenges and a far different political environment. In response, their priorities have shifted to meet the circumstances that different times have brought to their institutions.

But even as the current generation of leaders engages with their own priorities, the core issues of inequity in health care and the shortage of minority health practitioners continue to have a dire effect on the health of African Americans and other disadvantaged American communities. As the leadership baton passes from one generation to the next, the legislative tools and methods of utilizing combined power established over years of success are still available. The lessons of history are still available. The inspiration that derives from the African American legacy of community cohesion and mutual aid animates Black health leaders today—leaders who are fully capable of applying that energy and bringing new cures to our old, ingrained problems. In doing that, they will benefit not only their own community but will at the same time—if the past is any predictor—raise the health standards of the nation. I am encouraged and inspired by the talent and creativity of our current leaders, and I rest confident because of the successes they have had and the vision they bring to addressing the enduring challenges we continue to face as we move into the future.

LOUIS W. SULLIVAN, MD

ACKNOWLEDGMENTS

This book is a historical account that also looks to the future. In terms of the history, we've been able to draw on a variety of rich sources, prominent among them: the two volumes of *An American Health Dilemma* by Michael Byrd and Linda Clayton; Herbert Morais's classic work, *The History of the Negro in Medicine*; and the series of biographical profiles of Black physicians and medical scientists written by Montague Cobb, who for many years edited the *Journal of the National Medical Association*.

These and numerous other research sources offered a trove of data and interpretation, but we were especially fortunate to have been writing while many of the "early fathers" of the Association of Minority Health Professions Schools were still available to consult and interview. Among them we owe special gratitude to David Satcher, John Maupin, and Rueben Warren. David Satcher was one of the three school heads who accompanied Louis Sullivan in meeting with Health and Human Services Secretary Margaret Heckler, which precipitated the *Report of the Secretary's Task Force on Black and Minority Health*, the starting point for so much of the minority health legislation that came to fruition in the late 1980s and 1990s. John Maupin and Rueben Warren were intimately involved in the association's affairs (Maupin as president from 2001 to 2005), and both shared their experiences in ways crucial to telling the story, as did Dr. Satcher.

The phrase "without whom, nothing" is often used loosely. In the course of this project, though, there is one person whose contribution was absolutely essential to illuminating the legislative dance that brought the AMHPS-inspired political agenda to life and saw it through to success in both Republican and Democratic congresses. Dale Dirks of the Health and Medicine Counsel has been (and still is) the chief lobbyist for AMHPS, a role he took over from his father, Harley Dirks, in the early years of the association. Dale is the institutional memory of AMHPS. His commitment to getting this story told enabled our efforts in more ways than we have space to enumerate. A number of Dale's colleagues at the Health and Medicine Counsel helped research important but often difficult-to-find details and shared their own memories of people and events. We'd like to thank them for their help, in particular Lodriguez Murray, Joshua Lewis, Lesia Griffin, and Gavin Lindberg.

For part of this history, Ronny Lancaster (AMHPS president from 1998 to 2001) was Dale's full partner in working the levers of Congress. Ronny walked the halls with Dale and visited members of Congress and their staffs, gathering support for AMHPS's efforts to move critical bills through the daunting legislative obstacle course. Ronny was, in addition, the creative originator of some of AMHPS's most successful programs. His input, like Dale's, has been essential to our ability to reconstruct the association's history.

We also owe a debt of gratitude to John Ruffin, former director of NIH's National Institute on Minority Health and Health Disparities. John was director of the institute when it was first established as an NIH office in 1990. He provided strong leadership as it was elevated to an NIH center, and then to an institute. In his twenty-four years of service, he brought the facts of health disparities out of obscurity and denial into the light of scientific study and public awareness. His firsthand account of this evolution (struggle is perhaps a better term) was instrumental in illuminating the role played by AMHPS and its leaders in this process.

Another individual to whom we owe special thanks is Kenneth Ludmerer, one of today's preeminent medical historians. He read our manuscript with minute care, which saved us from various errors; his suggestions strengthened the book considerably. We are grateful to the Josiah Macy Jr. Foundation and the Association of Minority Health Professions Schools for their support. Others who gave their time to fill out parts of the AMHPS story or provide important background information include Thoru Pederson, Sidney McNairy, Barney Frank, Brian Smedley, Tony McAnn, Augustus White, Walter Sullivan, Donald Wilson, Rodney Whitlock, Shelley Stokes Hammond, Eric Hammond, Virginia Brennan, Elizabeth Ofili, Judy Miller Jones, Anna Mae Duane, Jessie Jackson Jr., Charles Dujon, Johnnie Early (dean of Florida A&M College of Pharmacy), Sandra Parham (Librarian Emerita, Meharry Medical College), and Kathleen Kennedy (dean of Xavier University College of Pharmacy and AMHPS's current president). Leslie Atkinson, Cheryl Smith, Fredette West, and Millicent Gorham, former staffers in Louis Stokes's congressional office, were instrumental in assembling the background data and arguments that went into the congressman's determined battle to right health care inequities. We thank them as well. We also want to remember Bud Blakey, whose career as a relentless advocate for Historically Black Colleges and Universities included originating the initial Title III legislation that served as a springboard, first for Morehouse School of Medicine funding and subsequently as a model for expanding support to other Black health institutions. Our thanks also go to Marybeth Gasman for her helpful advice regarding the publishing environment for books on Black medical history. We want to thank acquisitions assistant Adriahna Conway of Johns Hopkins University Press and copyeditor Susan Matheson for their hard, professional work in helping to bring our book through the production process. Our gratitude goes especially to our editor Robin Coleman for his wise and sympathetic guidance from inception through publication.

A final word about Congressman Louis Stokes, to whose memory we have dedicated this book. Through his thirty years in Congress, Lou Stokes exemplified service for the public good. He championed many good causes, but to none was he more dedicated than bettering the health of America's poor and underserved. Both of this book's authors were privileged to know him and work closely with him. He was on our minds continually as we wrote.

NOTES

Preface

1. Frederick Hoffman, *Race Traits and Tendencies of the American Negro*, 310; quoted in Beatrix Hoffman, "Scientific Racism, Insurance and Opposition to the Welfare State: Frederick Hoffman's Transatlantic Journey," *Journal of the Gilded Age and Progressive Era* 2, no. 2 (April 2003): 164.
2. Frederick Hoffman, *Race Traits and Tendencies of the American Negro*, 95; quoted in Megan J. Wolff, "The Myth of the Actuary: Life Insurance and Frederick L. Hoffman's *Race Traits and Tendencies of the American Negro*," *Public Health Reports* 121, no. 1 (January–February 2006): 84-91.
3. Frederick Hoffman, "Vital Statistics of the Negro," *Arena* 29 (April 1892): 529-42; quoted in William Darity Jr., "Many Roads to Extinction: Early AEA Economists and the Black Disappearance Hypothesis," *History of Economics Review* 21 no. 1 (1994): 47-64, https://doi.org/10.1080/10370196.1994.11733149.
4. W. E. B. Du Bois, "The Slaughter of the Innocents," editorial, *Crisis* 16, no. 6 (October 1918): 267.
5. W. Michael Byrd and Linda A. Clayton, *An American Health Dilemma: A Medical History of African Americans and the Problem of Race*, vol. 1, *Beginnings to 1900* (New York: Routledge, 2000), 398.

Chapter 1. The Nadir

1. Henry Stiles, *History and Genealogies of Ancient Windsor* (Hartford, CT: Lockwood & Brainard, 1891), 458.
2. Quoted in Herbert M. Morais, *The History of the Negro in Medicine*, vol. 3 of *International Library of Negro Life and History*, 5 vols. (New York: Publishers Company, 1967), 9.
3. Quoted in Dorothy Sterling, *The Making of an Afro-American: Martin Robison Delany, 1812-1885* (New York: Da Capo Press, 1996), 130.
4. Frederick Douglass, *North Star*, January 26, 1849.
5. Quoted in Sterling, *Making of an Afro-American*, 151.
6. "National Emigration Convention of Colored People," in *Encyclopedia of Cleveland History*, Case Western Reserve University, 1996, https://case.edu/ech/articles/n/national-emigration-convention-colored-people.
7. Anna Mae Duane, *Educated for Freedom* (New York: New York University Press, 2020), 156.

8. Sterling, *Making of an Afro-American*, 242.
9. Sterling, *Making of an Afro-American*, 243.
10. Martin Robison Delaney, *The Condition, Elevation, Emigration, and Destiny of the Colored People of the United States* (1852; Project Gutenberg, 2005), https://www.gutenberg.org/files/17154/17154-h/17154-h.htm.
11. Duane, *Educated for Freedom*, 35.
12. Ulysses Grant letter to sister Mary Grant, August 19, 1862; quoted in Donald Miller, *Vicksburg: Grant's Campaign That Broke the Confederacy* (New York: Simon & Schuster, 2019), 206.
13. Miller, *Vicksburg*, 206.
14. Levi Coffin, *Reminiscences of Levi Coffin* (Cincinnati: Robert Clarke, 1880), 621; quoted in Gaines M. Foster, "The Limitations of Federal Health Care for Freedmen, 1862–1868," *Journal of Southern History* 48, no. 3 (August 1982): 353.
15. W. Michael Byrd and Linda A. Clayton, *An American Health Dilemma: A Medical History of African Americans and the Problem of Race*, vol. 1, *Beginnings to 1900* (New York: Routledge, 2000), 329.
16. Morais, *History of the Negro in Medicine*, 5.
17. W. M. Cobb, "A Short History of Freedmen's Hospital," *Journal of the National Medical Association* 54, no. 3 (May 1962): 277.
18. Cobb, "Short History of Freedmen's Hospital," 277.
19. W. E. B. Du Bois, *Black Reconstruction in America* (New York: Free Press, 1935), 223.
20. US War Department, *Annual Report of the Secretary of War* (Washington, DC: US Government Printing Office, 1869).
21. Stephen J. Wright, "The Development of the Hampton-Tuskegee Pattern of Higher Education," *Phylon* 10, no 4 (1949): 334–42, https://doi.org/272114.
22. Morais, *History of the Negro in Medicine*, 52–58; Robert Baker, "The American Medical Association and Race," *AMA Journal of Ethics* 16, no. 6 (June 2014): 479–88.
23. Quoted in Morais, *History of the Negro in Medicine*, 53.
24. Quoted in Morais, *History of the Negro in Medicine*, 53.
25. Quoted in Morais, *History of the Negro in Medicine*, 39.
26. "Minutes of the 1870 AMA Convention," in Morais, *History of the Negro in Medicine*, appendix G, 218.

Chapter 2. The Response

1. Quoted in David McBride, *Caring for Equality* (New York: Rowman and Littlefield, 2018), 22.
2. Megan J. Wolff, "The Myth of the Actuary: Life Insurance and Frederick L. Hoffman's *Race Traits and Tendencies of the American Negro*," *Public Health Reports* 121, no. 1 (January–February 2006): 84–91.
3. John S. Billings, *Report on Mortality and Vital Statistics of the United States as Returned at the Tenth Census (June 1, 1880), Part 1* (Washington, DC:

Government Printing Office, 1885), https://www.census.gov/library /publications/1885/dec/vol-11-12-mortality.html.

4. McBride, *Caring for Equality*, 22.
5. Douglas Ewbank, "History of Black Mortality and Health before 1940," *Milbank Quarterly* 65, supplement 1 (1987): 106.
6. Ewbank, "History of Black Mortality," 116.
7. Todd Savitt, "Entering a White Profession: Black Physicians in the New South, 1880–1920," *Bulletin of the History of Medicine* 61, no. 4 (Winter 1987): 511.
8. Joycelyn Elders, *Joycelyn Elders, MD* (New York: William Morrow, 1996): 27.
9. W. Michael Byrd and Linda A. Clayton, *An American Health Dilemma: A Medical History of African Americans and the Problem of Race*, vol. 1, *Beginnings to 1900* (New York: Routledge, 2000), 389.
10. Louis W. Sullivan, *Missing Persons: Minorities in the Health Professions; A Report of the Sullivan Commission on Diversity in the Healthcare Workforce*, Digital Repository at the University of Maryland, 2004, https://doi.org/10 .13016/cwij-acxl.
11. Byrd and Clayton, *American Health Dilemma*, 390.
12. Wayne Riley, "The History of America's Premier Independent Black Medical School," *Journal of Blacks in Higher Education* 60 (Summer 2008): 74.
13. John H. Wilkins address before the Dallas meeting of the Lone Star State Medical, Dental, and Pharmaceutical Association, October 21, 1911; published in J. H. Wilkins, "History of the Lone Star State Medical, Dental, and Pharmaceutical Association," *Journal of the National Medical Association* 4, no. 1 (January–March 1912): 87–89.
14. Byrd and Clayton, *American Health Dilemma*, 394.
15. Montague Cobb, "Robert Fulton Boyd," *Journal of the National Medical Association* 45, no. 3 (May 1953): 233.
16. Quoted in Herbert M. Morais, *The History of the Negro in Medicine*, vol. 3 of *International Library of Negro Life and History*, 5 vols. (New York: Publishers Company, 1967), 80.
17. Robert Press, "In His Own Words: Nathan Francis Mossell, Penn Medicine's First Black Graduate," *Penn Medicine News*, blog, February 6, 2017. https://www.pennmedicine.org/news/news-blog/2017/february/in-his -own-words-nathan-francis-mossell.
18. Press, "In His Own Words."
19. N. F. Mossell, *Autobiographical Writings*; quoted in Vidya Viswanathan, "Medicine's Uncompromising Champion of Racial Justice," *Pharos*, Autumn 2018, https://www.alphaomegaalpha.org/wp-content/uploads /2021/03/2018-4-Viswanathan.pdf.
20. Byrd and Clayton, *American Health Dilemma*, 329.
21. Viswanathan, "Medicine's Uncompromising Champion," 5–6.
22. Montague Cobb, "Nathan Francis Mossell, MD, 1856–1946," *Journal of the National Medical Association* 46, no. 2 (March 1954): 122.

23. Wilkins, "History of the Lone Star State Medical, Dental, and Pharmaceutical Association."

24. Wilkins, "History of the Lone Star State Medical, Dental, and Pharmaceutical Association."

25. Miles V. Lynk, *Sixty Years of Medicine* (Memphis: Twentieth Century Press, 1951); quoted in Morais, *History of the Negro in Medicine*, 64.

26. Quoted in Morais, *History of the Negro in Medicine*, 68.

27. Byrd and Clayton, *American Health Dilemma*, 402.

Chapter 3. Abraham Flexner and the Black Medical Schools

1. Karen Morris, "The Founding of the National Medical Association" (medical thesis, Yale School of Medicine, 2007), 82, Yale Medicine Thesis Digital Library, https://elischolar.library.yale.edu/ymtdl/360.

2. Quoted in Barry D. Silverman, "William Henry Welch (1850–1934): The Road to Johns Hopkins," *Baylor University Medical Center Proceedings* 24, no. 3 (July 2011): 236–42, https://doi.org/10.1080/08998280.2011.11928722.

3. John Duffy, *From Humors to Medical Science: A History of American Medicine*, 2nd ed. (Urbana: University of Illinois Press, 1993), 168.

4. William Welch, "Some of the Conditions Which Have Influenced the Development of American Medicine," 1908; quoted in Silverman, "William Henry Welch."

5. Kenneth Ludmerer, *Learning to Heal* (Baltimore: Johns Hopkins University Press, 1985), 57.

6. Paul Starr, *The Social Transformation of American Medicine* (New York: Basic Books 1982), 115.

7. Martin Kaufman, "Edward H. Dixon and Medical Education in New York," *New York History* 51, no. 4 (July 1970): 399.

8. Quoted in W. Michael Byrd and Linda A. Clayton, *An American Health Dilemma*, vol. 2, *Race, Medicine, and Health Care in the United States, 1900–2000* (New York: Routledge, 2002), 94.

9. Ludmerer, *Learning to Heal*, 168.

10. Ludmerer, *Learning to Heal*, 67, 68.

11. Starr, *Social Transformation*, 119.

12. Henry S. Pritchett, introduction to Abraham Flexner, *Medical Education in the United States and Canada: A Report to the Carnegie Foundation for the Advancement of Teaching* [known as the Flexner Report], 1910, 3.

13. Starr, *Social Transformation*, 120.

14. Donald Fleming, *William H. Welch and the Rise of Modern Medicine* (Boston: Little, Brown, 1954), 179.

15. Thomas Duffy, "The Flexner Report—100 Years Later," *Yale Journal of Biology and Medicine* 84, no. 3 (September 2011): 269–76.

16. Quoted in Starr, *Social Transformation*, 125.

17. Rosemary Stevens, *American Medicine and the Public Interest* (New Haven, CT: Yale University Press, 1971), 68; quoted in Byrd and Clayton, *American Health Dilemma*, vol. 2, 95.

Chapter 4. AMHPS: The Founding

1. Harry Truman, "President Truman's Address before the NAACP," June 29, 1947, Truman Library Institute, https://www.trumanlibraryinstitute.org /historic-speeches-naacp/.
2. Press conference March 25, 1966, prior to King's address to the annual meeting of the Medical Committee for Human Rights, Chicago.

Chapter 5. The Heckler Report

1. John Ruffin, *Going the Distance: The Making of a National Health Disparities Research Enterprise* (Chicago: Hilton, 2015), 5.
2. W. Michael Byrd and Linda A. Clayton, *An American Health Dilemma*, vol. 2, *Race, Medicine, and Health Care in the United States, 1900–2000* (Routledge, New York, 2002), 521.
3. Louis Stokes, *The Gentleman from Ohio* (Columbus: Ohio State University Press, 2016), 211.

Chapter 7. AMHPS and the Secretary

1. Louis Stokes, *The Gentleman from Ohio* (Columbus: Ohio State University Press, 2016), 235.
2. Stokes, *Gentleman from Ohio*, 222.
3. Stokes, *Gentleman from Ohio*, 127.
4. Sidney McNairy, in discussion with David Chanoff, July 8, 2020.
5. Louis Sullivan, *Breaking Ground* (Athens: University of Georgia Press, 2014), 126.
6. Sullivan, *Breaking Ground*, 127.
7. Barbara Bush, in discussion with David Chanoff, October 5, 2013.
8. Marybeth Gasman, *The Morehouse Mystique* (Baltimore: Johns Hopkins University Press, 2012), 86.

Chapter 8. The Office of Minority Health

1. Dale Dirks, in discussion with David Chanoff, July 28, 2020.
2. Louis Stokes, *The Gentleman from Ohio* (Columbus: Ohio State University Press, 2016), 224.
3. John Ruffin, in discussion with David Chanoff, August 5, 2020.
4. John Ruffin, *Going the Distance: The Making of a National Health Disparities Research Enterprise* (Chicago: Hilton, 2015), 17.
5. Dale Dirks, in discussion with David Chanoff, August 12, 2020.
6. Ruffin, *Going the Distance*, xi.
7. Dale Dirks, in discussion with David Chanoff, July 28, 2020.
8. John Ruffin, in discussion with David Chanoff, July 5, 2020.

Chapter 9. The Center for Minority Health and Health Disparities

1. Louis Stokes, *The Gentleman from Ohio* (Columbus: Ohio State University Press, 2016, 225.
2. Stokes, *Gentleman from Ohio*, 226.

3. Dale Dirks, in discussion with David Chanoff, August 12, 2020.
4. Dirks, discussion.
5. Eric T. Rosenthal, "Michael Link, ASCO's First Pediatric Oncologist President, Looks Back and to the Future," *Oncology Times* 33, no. 10 (May 25, 2011): 13–14.
6. Quoted in Associated Press, "The Speaker Steps Down," *New York Times*, November 8, 1998, section 1, page 24.
7. US Senate Subcommittee on Departments of Labor, Health and Human Services, and Education, and Related Agencies, hearing, January 21, 1999, 25.

Chapter 10. A National Institute

1. Quoted in John Ruffin, *Going the Distance: The Making of a National Health Disparities Research Enterprise* (Chicago: Hilton, 2015), 65.
2. John Maupin, in discussion with David Chanoff, October 2, 2020.
3. Joycelyn Elders, *Joycelyn Elders, MD* (New York: William Morrow, 1996), 230.
4. Ruffin, *Going the Distance*, 54.
5. Ruffin, *Going the Distance*, 56.
6. US Department of Health and Human Services, *Report of the Secretary's Task Force on Black and Minority Health*, August 1985, 5. See also David Satcher, George E. Fryer Jr., Jessica McCann, Adewale Troutman, Steven H. Woolf, and George Rust, "What If We Were Equal? A Comparison of the Black-White Mortality Gap in 1960 and 2000," *Health Affairs* 24, no. 2 (March/April 2005): 459–64.
7. See Augustus White and David Chanoff, *Seeing Patients* (Cambridge, MA: Harvard University Press, 2011), 211.
8. Brian D. Smedley, Adrienne Y. Stith, and Alan R. Nelson, eds., *Unequal Treatment: Confronting Racial and Ethnic Disparities in Healthcare* (Washington, DC: Institute of Medicine, 2003), 5, 6.
9. White and Chanoff, *Seeing Patients*, 213.
10. Louis Sullivan, *Breaking Ground* (Athens: University of Georgia Press, 2014), 77–80.
11. Donna K. Ginther, Walter T. Schaffer, Joshua Schnell, Beth Masimore, Faye Liu, Laurel L. Haak, and Raynard Kington, "Race, Ethnicity, and NIH Research Awards," *Science* 333, no. 6045 (August 19, 2011): 1015–19. Although published in 2011, the study was based on NIH data from 2000 to 2006.
12. Louis Sullivan, in discussion with David Chanoff, September 19, 2021.
13. Dale Dirks, in discussion with David Chanoff, September 21, 2020.
14. Francis Collins's conversation reconstructed from memories of several people in the room.

Chapter 11. A Common Mission

1. John Ruffin, *Going the Distance: The Making of a National Health Disparities Research Enterprise* (Chicago: Hilton, 2015), 162.

2.   Ronny Lancaster, in discussion with David Chanoff, September 22, 2020.

3.   Walter Sullivan, in discussion with David Chanoff, October 25, 2020.

4.   Rueben Warren, in discussion with David Chanoff, October 26, 2020.

5.   APM Research Lab Report, "The Color of Coronavirus: COVID-19 Deaths by Race and Ethnicity in the US," https://www.apmresearchlab.org/covid/deaths-by-race, data from October 15, 2020. Age-adjusted rates take account of age distributions when comparing distinct communities. Age adjustment is considered the most accurate way to judge comparisons.

6.   David Satcher, George E. Fryer Jr., Jessica McCann, Adewale Troutman, Steven H. Woolf, and George Rust, "What If We Were Equal? A Comparison of the Black-White Mortality Gap in 1960 and 2000," *Health Affairs* 24, no. 2 (March/April 2005): 459–64.

7.   John Ruffin, in discussion with David Chanoff, August 5, 2020.

8.   Ruffin, discussion.

9.   Fitzhugh Mullan, Candice Chen, Stephen Petterson, Gretchen Kolsky, and Michael Spagnola, "The Social Mission of Education: Ranking the Schools," *Annals of Internal Medicine* 152, no. 12 (June 15, 2010): 804–11.

10. Warren, discussion.

11. Mullan et al., "Social Mission of Education."

12. Walter Sullivan, in discussion with David Chanoff, October 17, 2020.

INDEX

AAMC (Association of American Medical Colleges), 206
AAMP (Association for Academic Minority Physicians), 191
Advanced Financial Distress Program, 92, 93–94
affirmative action, 106
Affordable Care Act (ACA), 186, 188–89
African Americans: Black physicians and health practitioners, shortage of (1970s), xvii–xviii; health disparities in 19th century, xv–xvii; Hoffman's extinction thesis, xv–xvi, 20; lack of medical care (1895), xvii; population growth, 1900–1910, xvi. *See also* mortality and morbidity, African American; *and Black terms*
African Methodist Episcopal (AME) Church, 13
Agnew, David Hays, 29, 31
AIDS, as priority for Sullivan, 124
Alcorn State University, 13
American College, The (Flexner), 43
American Economic Association, ix
American Medical Association (AMA): Black health care, destructive impact of AMA discrimination on, 16–17; prohibition of segregation in local medical societies (1968), 17; push for professional standards for medical education, 43; racial discrimination within, 15–17
American Missionary Association, 22
AMHPS. *See* Association of Minority Health Professions Schools (AMHPS)
Association for Academic Minority Physicians (AAMP), 191
Association of American Medical Colleges (AAMC), 206

Association of Minority Health Professions Schools (AMHPS): access to government agencies, 125–26; addressing specific health problems, 217; biomedical symposia of, 193–96, 202; bipartisan legislative strategies, 103–4, 105, 126–27, 165–66; "Black lives matter" as central theme, 200; as catalyst in minority health, 201–2; concerns for future, 215; congressional allies, 65, 149–50; Contract with America impact on, 147; dearth of minority physicians as motivating force, 182; declining activism of, 191, 197; dedication ceremony for first independent Morehouse building, 113–15; delayed follow-up by Heckler to meeting with, 74–76; elevating NCMHD to National Institute, 185–89; elevating Office of Research on Minority Health to NIH Center, 153–55; expanding advocacy to underserved non-minorities, 172, 207; focus on keeping legislation funded, 109, 113; founding of, xviii–xix, 63–64, 213; funding for "historically Black" institutions under Title III of Higher Education Act, 87–89; hiring Washington lobbyist and other staff, 67–68; importance recognized by Dirks at National Health Council meeting, 124–25; inability of minority schools to compete for funding with major institutions, 203; incorporation of, 66–67; inherent strength of, 201; institutional challenges for current leadership, 218; integration of faculties, 113;

Association of Minority Health Professions Schools (AMHPS) (*continued*) leadership, changing priorities of, 184–85; leading issues for, 203; legislative achievements in 1980s, 101–2; mainstreaming health disparities issues, 191; membership and institutional collaboration, 213–14; as national catalyst on minority health issues, 108; need for member institutions to return to united action, 201–2; new roles for, 207–8; non-African American communities, embracing, 208–9; origin and maturation of, 107–8; punching above its weight, 202, 215; racial inequities in health care, addressing, xxii, 67; renewing cross-institutional ties, 202; Republican administrations and success of initiatives, 165; rotation of presidency among schools, 108; Ruffin's relationship with, 136; social mission of minority schools, 205–6; social/political change and organization of, 212–13; successes and power of collaboration, 214; timeline, xxiii–xxiv; *Unequal Treatment* as playbook, 178; White Paper on African American health care resources, xvi–xx

Atlanta Baptist College, 56
Atlanta Clark University, 13
Atlanta University, 55
Atlanta University Center Consortium, 55, 108
Augusta, Alexander T., 11, 13–14

Back to Africa movement, 3
bacteria, discovery of, 40
Battle of Fort Sumter (1861), 5
Battle of Seven Pines, 10
Bennett, Bill, 48, 122
Black, Keith, 195
Black education, Freedmen's Bureau and, 12, 13
Black Hospital Movement, 28
Black Lives Matter movement, 198–99, 207, 211
Black physicians, in Revolutionary period, 1–2

"Blacks and the Health Professions in the '80s: A National Crisis and a Time for Action" (Hanft), 69–70, 82, 133, 198
Blakely, GA, lack of health care providers in, 53
Blakey, William "Bud," 87
Bob Jones University, 114
Bond, Julian, 49, 115
Boner, Bill, 95
Booker, Cory, xxi
Boren, David, 105
Boston University, 51
Bowie, Walter: Excellence in Minority Health Education and Care Act and, 94; as founding member of AMHPS, 63; keynote speaker at first biomedical symposium, 194; participation in AMHPS presentation to Heckler, xix, 73–74; retirement of, 184; at Tuskegee, 76, 194
Boyd, Robert: born into plantation slavery, 36; early education of, 36; as first Black doctor/dentist in Nashville, 37; as foremost Black physician of his day, 38; founding Mercy Hospital in Nashville as Meharry teaching hospital, 37; medical/dental education at Meharry, 36–37; as NMA founding member and first president, 33, 34, 37; as physician and dentist, 25
Brain Trusts, 64–65, 82, 83, 127
Braveman, Paula, 190–91
Brown, Louis, 59
Bush, Barbara: attending Sullivan's swearing in as HHS secretary, 121; friendship with Sullivan, 116; joining Morehouse School of Medicine board of directors, 116
Bush, George H. W.: philanthropy toward Black organizations, 116; positive race relations of, 115–16; social friendship with William Trent, 116; speaking at Morehouse building dedication ceremony, 115
Bush, George W., 165
Byrd, Robert, 170–73, 208

Cardin, Ben, 188-89
Cardiovascular Research Institute,
	Morehouse School of Medicine, 113
*Carnegie Foundation Bulletin Number
	Four. See* Flexner Report (1910)
Carnegie Foundation for the Advance-
	ment of Teaching, 43
Carson, Ben, 195
Carver, George Washington, 94
CBC. *See* Congressional Black Caucus
	(CBC)
cell theory of disease, 39
Centers for Disease Control and
	Prevention (CDC), 85
Centers for Excellence in Minority
	Health program: AMHPS cam-
	paign to elevate to National
	Institute, 185-89; planning for
	health disparities research across
	all NIH centers and institutes,
	173-75; reauthorization of, 130
Centers of Excellence programs (NIH),
	as funding mechanism, 168-70
Central Tennessee College, Meharry
	Medical Department (Nashville),
	22
Charles R. Drew Postgraduate Medical
	School, 64, 213
Charles R. Drew University of Medicine
	and Science, xviii, 169
Cheney State College (Pennsylvania), 13
Civil Rights Act (1964), 56-57, 198
civil rights movement: changing
	nation's mindset on equality, 106;
	effects on medical schools, 180;
	key events shaping, 56-57; Mays as
	one of founders, 49
Civil War, US: abolition of slavery, 7;
	mortality rates among former
	slaves, 8-9; refugee crisis of, 7-8
Claremont College Consortium, 54
Clark College, 55
Clay, William, 65, 90, 106
clinical trials, insufficient women
	enrolled in, 123
Clinton, Bill, 136, 183
Cobb, Montague, 25
Cochran, Thad, 105
Collins, Francis, 187-88
Columbia University College of
	Physicians and Surgeons, 38

*Condition, Elevation, Emigration, and
	Destiny of the Colored People of the
	United States, The* (Delany), 4, 6
Congressional Black Caucus (CBC),
	xxii, 64, 106, 107, 127
Conte, Silvio, 104
Contract with America, 141, 143, 144, 147
Cotton, Ray, 68, 114-15
Cotton States and International
	Exposition (Atlanta, 1885), 33
COVID-19 pandemic: Black inequality
	and, 199-200; death rates and hos-
	pitalizations, Black vs. white rates,
	xxi; health disparities, African
	American, xxi, 211; minority health
	professions schools and, 215; spot-
	lighting health inequalities, 84-85

Dannemeyer, William, 96-97
Davis, Nathan Smith, 16
De Grasse, John, 31
Delany, Martin Robison: emigration
	ending friendship with Smith, 5;
	emigration movement, support for,
	3-6; forced disenrollment from
	Harvard Medical School, 2; inter-
	view with Abraham Lincoln, 5;
	organizing National Emigration
	Convention of Colored People
	(Cleveland, 1854), 4; as partner
	with Douglass in *The North Star*, 5;
	photograph of (description), 4-5;
	proposing army of freed slaves to
	Abraham Lincoln, 5; rejecting infe-
	riority of Blacks, 4; as surgeon to
	Black Union troops, 5
Derham, James (Black physician), 1-2
Dillard University, 13
Dirks, Dale: amendment to ACA
	elevating National Center to
	National Institute, 187-89; on
	AMHPS relationship with Ruffin,
	136; campaign to elevate Office
	of Research on Minority Health
	to NIH Center, 153-55; as chief
	lobbyist for AMHPS, 91, 109, 124,
	183; on Contract with America
	impact on AMHPS, 147; Excellence
	in Minority Health Education and
	Care Act and, 94; on Ruffin and
	conflicts within NIH, 139

Dirks, Harley, 91
Disadvantaged Minority Health
    Improvement Act (1990),
    128-30
Dole, Bob, 180
Dotson, Betty Lou, 77
Douglass, Frederick: on emigration
    movement, 3; *My Bondage and My
    Freedom*, 6; relationship with
    Smith, 6
Dow, Robert, 1
Duane, Anna Mae, 4
Du Bois, W. E. B.: criticism of Hoff-
    man's *Race Traits*, xvi; on Freed-
    men's Bureau responsibilities, 11;
    Hope as associate of, 54
Duffy, John, 38-39
Duffy, Thomas, 46

education, medical: American,
    scientific basis missing for, in late
    19th century, 38; barriers for Black
    students, late 19th century, xvii;
    Flexner Report and closure of
    most Black and women's schools,
    47; physician shortage and
    expansion of, 212-13. *See also*
    schools, medical
Elam, Lloyd, 62-63
Elders, Joycelyn, 19-20, 173
Emancipation Proclamation, 7
emigration movement, pre–Civil War:
    Delany's advocacy of, 3-5;
    Douglass on, 3; Smith's rejection
    of, 6-7
endowments: for Black medical
    schools, 154-55; research endow-
    ments, 166-67
Eve, Paul, 36
Excellence in Minority Health
    Education and Care Act, 91-98;
    amendments covering Hispanic-
    and Native American–serving
    institutions, 97-98; amendments
    folding in other AMHPS institu-
    tions, 97; as amendment to Public
    Health Service Act, Title VII, 94;
    legislative hearings and passage
    of, 95-97, 206; NIH Health
    Revitalization Act and, 136-37

FDA (Food and Drug Administration),
    85
First Congregational Society, Washing-
    ton, DC, 12
Fisk University, 13
Flexner, Abraham, 36-47; *American
    College, The*, 43; as educator and
    reformer, xvii, 43; evaluation of
    medical schools based on teaching
    methods and graduation stan-
    dards, 26, 44-45; Johns Hopkins
    program as model for medical
    education, 44; on "The Medical
    Education of the Negro," 47.
    See also Flexner Report (1910)
Flexner, Simon, 43
Flexner Report (1910): criticism of
    scientific emphasis in, 46; impact
    on Black medical schools, xvii, 26,
    45, 54; inadequacies of US/
    Canadian medical schools, 45, 54;
    incorporating biosciences into
    medical school curricula, 44;
    "Medical Education of the Negro,
    The," 47; as most significant
    document in American health care,
    46
Flint Medical College, 26, 47
Florida A&M University: College of
    Pharmacy, xviii, 25, 64; dental
    school, 25
Floyd, George, murder of, 199, 211
folk healers, 53
Food and Drug Administration (FDA),
    85
Fort Sumter, Battle of (1861), 5
Foster, Henry, 50
Fourteenth Amendment to Constitu-
    tion, 7
Francis, Norman, 63, 95, 134
Frank, Barney, 85
Frederick Douglass Memorial Hospital
    and Training School (Philadel-
    phia), 28, 29
Freedmen's Aid Society, 22
Freedmen's Bureau: Black education
    and, 12; closure in 1872, 10-11;
    responsibilities of, 10-11; schools
    established by, 21-22
Freedmen's Hospital, 11-12, 13, 20

Friedrich Wilhelm University (Berlin), 39
Frist, Bill: as congressional champion for minority health, xxi; supporting Minority Health and Health Disparities Research and Education Act, 156–57, 163
Fugitive Slave Law (1850), 3

Galletti, Pierre, 48
Gayles, Joseph, 48, 51
George Washington University School of Medicine and Health Sciences: NIH funding inversely associated with social justice scores, 206; social justice rankings of medical schools, 205–6
Georgia: African American morbidity and mortality, 1970s, 50; shortage of Black health care providers, 50, 53
germ theory of disease, 40
Gibbons, Garry, 113
Gingrich, Newt: banning personal contact between Republican and Democratic House members, 146; Contract with America, 141, 143, 144; health-related budget cuts under, 144–45; as House minority whip, 142; loss of speakership, 150–51; loyalty oath on Republican House members, 146; as Morehouse supporter, 142; partial protection for NIH and Black medical schools, 150; political trench warfare of, 143; promoting toxic partisanship of Congress, 145; relationship with Sullivan, 142–43; as Speaker of the House, 141, 144
Ginther, Donna, 182, 191
Gloster, Hugh: Black equality as incentive for Morehouse medical school, 57; efforts to launch medical school at Morehouse, 48–50, 56; on windows of opportunity for funding of new medical school, 58
Going the Distance (Ruffin), 174
Grace, Marcellus, 94

Grant, Ulysses, 7
Great Society, 123
Griffin, Joseph, 53

Halsted, Stewart, 41
Hampton University, 25
Hanft, Ruth, 67, 68–69
Hanft Report. *See* "Blacks and the Health Professions in the '80s: A National Crisis and a Time for Action" (Hanft)
Harkin, Tom, xxi, 130
Harvard Medical School, 2, 181
Hatfield, Mark, 88, 104
Haverty, Rhodes, 59
Hayes, Barbara, 184
Haynes, Alfred: Drew School of Medicine and, 76; participation in AMHPS presentation to Heckler, xix, 73–74; retirement of, 184; testimony on insufficient NCI funding for minority issues, 152, 192
HBCU (Historically Black Colleges and Universities), 195, 213
Health and Medicine Counsel (lobbying firm), 68
Health Brain Trust, 64–65, 83, 127
Health Careers Opportunity Program, 129
Health Care Financing Administration (HCFA), Bill Toby as head of, 122
health disparities: African Americans in 19th century, ix; AMHPS promoting awareness of, 210; COVID-19 pandemic and, xix–xx, xxi, 199–200; Heckler Report introduction and, 79–80, 210; as legacy of segregation, 57; Office of Minority Affairs addressing, 132–33; political landscape and recognition of, 65–66; recognizing power of combined voices, 216–17; severity of minority health issues, xxi; shortage of Black health care providers, xvii–xviii, 57, 198, 210; strategic plan on, NCMHD, 167; timeline, xxiii–xxiv; unavailability of health care for Blacks in rural South, 19
Healy, Bernadine, 122, 123

Heckler, Margaret: AMHPS presentation on health disparities to,
xix–xx, 73–74; appointment of
task force to investigate health
disparities of minorities, 76–78;
awareness of inadequate number
of Black students in medical
schools, 72; establishment of
Office of Minority Health (1985),
84; forced out as HHS secretary
following release of Report, 85;
as HHS secretary under Reagan,
70–71; on importance of Report
for challenging health disparities,
79–80; as moderate misfit in Reagan administration, 85–86
Heckler Report (*Report of the Secretary's
Task Force on Black and Minority
Health*, 1985): asserting American
obligation to care for health of
Black and minority populations,
168, 210; condemning Reagan
health care–related funding cuts,
81; distribution and legislative
successes of, xix–xx; Malone's
letter explaining significance of,
78–79; meeting with AMHPS
precipitating, xx, 86; scope
exceeding expectations of AMHPS,
80–81; timeline for producing, 78
HHS. *See* US Health and Human
Services Department (HHS)
Higginbotham, Leon, 121
Hildreth, James, 113
Historically Black Colleges and
Universities (HBCU), 195, 213
Hoffman, Frederick: Du Bois's criticism
of *Race Traits*, x; extinction thesis,
xv–xvi; morbidity and mortality
statistics, xv; *Race Traits and
Tendencies of the American Negro*,
xv–xvi; racism of extinction
projections, xvi–xvii, 20
Hope, John: as first Black president of
Morehouse, 54, 55; foundation of
Niagara Movement and, 54; as
president of Atlanta University, 56
Hopkins, Donald, 77
Howard, Oliver Otis: on Black educa-
tion, 12; as "Christian General," 10,
12; founding of Howard University,

12; Freedmen's Bureau and, 10–11;
military career, 10
Howard Normal and Theological
Institute for the Education of
Preachers and Teachers, 12
Howard University: center of excellence
designation, 169; dental school, 24;
diverse and cosmopolitan nature of,
21; Flexner Report (1910) on, xvii,
47; founding of, 12, 213; Freedmen's
Hospital as teaching hospital, 13;
governmental affiliation of, 21;
medical department, establishment of (1867), 13, 20; Meharry
Medical College vs., 23–24; minority and female graduates of, 21;
pharmacy department, 25
Hubbard, George Whipple, 23
humors (physiology), 39
Humphries, Frederick, 90
Hunt, Harriet Kezia, 2

immunology, 40
Institute of Medicine (IOM), 151
Institutions of Emerging Excellence, 137

Jackson, Jesse, Jr., 157
Jackson, Marque, 56
Jackson, Maynard, 49, 115
Jemison, Mae, 195
Johns Hopkins School of Medicine:
biomedical model of, 26; curricu-
lum and educational reforms,
41–42; Welch as founding dean and
first professor, 40–41
Johnston, J. Bennett, 95
Joint Center for Political and Economic
Studies, 106–7
Jones, Judy Miller, 70
*Journal of Health Care for the Poor and
Underserved*, 202–3

Kelly, Howard, 41
Kennedy, Ted, xxi, 83, 95
King, Gwendolyn, 122
King, Martin Luther, Jr.: civil rights
movement and assassination of,
50, 57, 106, 198; inequality and
injustice in health of African
Americans, 57, 72–73, 180; Mays
as mentor of, 49

Kirschstein, Ruth, 130, 136, 201
Klausner, Richard, 152
"Know Nothings," Congressional,
     149
Knoxville Medical College, 47
Koop, C. Everett, 117

Lancaster, Ronny: campaign to elevate
     Office of Research on Minority
     Health to NIH Center, 153–55, 166;
     ongoing advocacy for minority
     health, 184; as principal deputy
     assistant secretary, NIH, 122, 153
Landsteiner, Karl, 40
Leeuwenhoek, Antoni van, 40
legislation, minority health–related,
     84–102; Disadvantaged Minority
     Health Improvement Act (1990),
     128–30; Excellence in Minority
     Health Education and Care Act
     (Title VII), 91–98; Minority Health
     and Health Disparities Research
     and Education Act (2000), 163–64,
     166; NIH Health Revitalization Act
     (1993), 136–37; Research Centers in
     Minority Institutions (RCMI) Act
     (1986), 100–101, 192; Strengthen-
     ing Historically Black Graduate
     Institutions (Title III), 87–89, 91;
     Title III Higher Education Act,
     Part B, Section 326 (1978), 87–89
Leonard Medical College, 47
Lewis, Carol, 196
Lewis, Jerry (congressman, California),
     145–46
Lewis, John, 115
Liberian colonization, 3
life expectancy, Black males (1900), 18
life insurance, unavailability to Black
     Americans, 18
Lincoln, Abraham, 8
Lincoln Memorial University (Tennes-
     see), 12
Livingston, Bob, 144, 148
loan repayment programs: expansion
     to underserved nonminorities,
     170–73; minority faculty educa-
     tional loans, 129; Minority Health
     and Health Disparities Research
     and Education Act, 170–73
Loomis, Silas, 15–17

Louisville National Medical College, 26,
     47
Ludmerer, Kenneth, 41
Lynk, Myles Vandarhurst, 33

MacLeish, Peter, 113
Madigan, Edward, 130
Magnuson, Warren, xxi, 65
Malone, Thomas: chair, Task Force on
     Black and Minority Health, 76–77,
     175; introductory letter on signifi-
     cance of Heckler Report, 78–79,
     175
Manumit, Primus, 1, 2, 25
Marshall, Thurgood, 106
Massachusetts Medical Society, 31
Massey, J. Britton, 31
Mattingly, Matt, 105
Maupin, John, 172, 184
Mays, Benjamin, 49
McCormick, Cyrus, 28
McNairy, Sidney, 109–13, 204
Medical and Surgical Observer, The
     (Black journal), 33
medical science: Germany as acknowl-
     edged leader in 19th century, 39;
     neglect in American schools in
     19th century, 38
medical societies: African American,
     32–33; AMA prohibition of segrega-
     tion in (1968), 17; Massachusetts
     Medical Society accepting mem-
     bership of de Grasse, 31; Medical
     Society of the District of Columbia
     (MSDC), 13–14; National Medical
     Association (NMA), 34–35; Phila-
     delphia Medical Society accepting
     membership of Mossell, 31; racial
     discrimination of AMA, 15–17, 31
Medical Society of the District of
     Columbia (MSDC), 13–14
medical specialties, biased care in, 177
Meharry, Samuel, 22–23
Meharry Dental College, 24, 92
Meharry Medical College: Center of
     Excellence designation, 169; debt
     burden, 75–76; Elam as president,
     62–63; endowment funds (2020),
     167; Flexner Report on, xvii, 47;
     foundation story, 22–23; grants
     from Advanced Financial Distress

Meharry Medical College (*continued*)
  Program, 92; Howard University,
  differences from, 23–24; Mercy
  Hospital as teaching hospital, 37;
  as second Black medical school in
  US, 94–95, 213
mentoring programs for minority
  students, 191
Mercer School of Medicine, 61
Metcalf, Ralph, 65
miasma theory of disease, 39
minority faculty educational loan
  repayment program, 129
Minority Health, Office of. *See* Office of
  Research on Minority Health
Minority Health and Health Disparities
  Research and Education Act
  (2000): bipartisan support for,
  158–59, 166; Democratic sponsors,
  157; drafting of, 155–56; endowments of Black medical schools,
  154–55; expansion of loan repayment programs to underserved
  nonminorities, 170–73; gathering
  support for, 156–59; "hold" on bill
  by unnamed senator, 162–63; opposition by NIH director Harold
  Varmus, 159–62; signing of, 163–64
minority health professions schools:
  COVID-19 pandemic and, 215;
  rebuilding trust in medical
  establishment, 216; recognizing
  power of combined voices, 216–17
*Missing Persons: Minorities in the Health
  Professions*, 179
Morais, Herbert, 9
Morehouse College: Gloster's campaign
  to create medical school at, 48–50;
  as historically Black college, 13;
  strengths of, 49
Morehouse Neuroscience Institute, 113
Morehouse School of Medicine: center
  of excellence designation, 169; cooperation with Mercer in seeking
  capitation funding, 61; dedication
  ceremony for first independent
  building, 113–15; endowment funds
  (2020), 167; funding of start-up
  programs, xviii, 75; "hold harmless" agreement assuring stability
  of Section 326 funding for, 89–91;

launch of, 60, 213; NMA concerns
  about federal funding, 60; obtaining funding as "historically Black"
  medical school, 87–88; separation
  from college, 75; Sullivan as founding dean, 50–52; transition to four-
  year school, 87–88
Morris Brown College, 55
Morrison, Toni, 183
mortality and morbidity, African American: COVID-19 pandemic and, xxi,
  199–200; Emancipation and, 27;
  among former slaves, 8–9; in Georgia, 1970s, 50; Hanft report documenting, 74; Heckler Report wid-
  ening scope of health disparities to
  other groups, 81; Hoffman's racism
  and, xvi–xvii, xxi, 20; infant mortality, xvii, 216; as legacy of segregation, 57; post–Civil War, 18–19;
  "What If We Were Equal? A Comparison of the Black-White Mortality Gap in 1960 and 2000," *Health
  Affairs* (Satcher et al.), 200
Mossell, Nathan Francis, 28–29, 30, 31
Mullan, Fitzhugh, 206
Murray, Lodriguez, 188
My Bondage and My Freedom (Douglass), 6

Natcher, William, 104
National Association for the Advance-
  ment of Colored People (NAACP),
  6, 54
National Cancer Institute (NCI), 151–52
National Center for Bioethics in
  Research and Health Care
  (Tuskegee University), 197
National Center for Nursing Research,
  130
National Center for Primary Care
  (Morehouse School of Medicine),
  208
National Center for Research Resources,
  101
National Center on Minority Health
  and Health Disparities (NCMHD):
  Affordable Care Act amendment
  elevating NCMHD to National In-
  stitute, 187–89; centers of excel-
  lence designations by, 169–70;

grant awards, 167; key provisions, 167–68; legislation establishing, 155–56, 166; loan repayment programs, 167, 170–73; research endowments, 166–67; strategic plan on health care disparities, 167

National Council of Colored People, 6

National Emigration Convention of Colored People (Cleveland, 1854), 4

National Health Council, Sullivan's keynote address to, 124

National Health Service Corps scholarship program, 75

National Human Genome Research Institute, 137, 187

National Institute of General Medical Sciences, 194

National Institute on Deafness, 130

National Institute on Minority Health and Health Disparities (NIMHD): budget limitations, 174–75; NIH resistance to mission of, 190; research support of, 214; significance of elevation from National Center, 190

National Institutes of Health (NIH): barriers to health disparities research, 173–75; Bernadine Healy as first female director, 122; funding of medical research, 70; grant proposals review process, 138–39; Health Revitalization Act (1993), 136–37; insufficient funding for minority scientists, 161; minority researchers sidetracked by, 191; neglect of health of minorities prior to Heckler Report, 85; P-50 research program grants, 191; political support for, 130; RCMI administration under, 101

National Medical Association (NMA), 34–35, 37

National Medical Society of the District of Columbia (NMS), 14–17

NCI (National Cancer Institute), 151–52

NCMHD. *See* National Center on Minority Health and Health Disparities (NCMHD)

Nelson, Alan, 178

New York Genome Center, 162

Niagara Movement, 54

NIH. *See* National Institutes of Health (NIH)

NIMHD. *See* National Institute on Minority Health and Health Disparities (NIMHD)

NMA (National Medical Association), 34–35, 37

Norris, Keith, 113

North Star, The (newspaper), 3, 5

Norwood, Charlie, 157

Novello, Antonia, 122

Nunn, Sam, 65

nursing schools, Black, 27–28

Obama, Barack, 100, 186

Office of House Legislative Counsel, 148

Office of Research on Minority Health: cultural gap within NIH, 138–39; deputy assistant secretary of HHS leading, 84–85, 86; disadvantages for AMHPS researchers in obtaining NIH funding, 139; establishment of (1985), 84; fact-finding committee recommendations, 134; limited resources of, 133; mission of, 132; as orphan agency within NIH, 137–38; political threats to, 136; racism affecting grant proposals, 140; Ruffin as director, 131–32; Sullivan's push for elevation to NIH Center status, 152; upgrade to Center in 2000, 139

O'Neill, Tip, 83

organizations, life cycle of, 211

Osler, William, 41, 46

Packwood, Robert, 104

Pasteur, Louis, 40

Penn, Garland, 33, 34

Philadelphia Medical Society, 31

Porter, John Edward: as advocate for medical research, 149; as chair of Labor H subcommittee, 144, 148–49; fighting back against Gingrich, 149; as founder of Congressional Human Rights Caucus, 148; leading legislative battles, xxi; protective stance toward Black medical schools, 149–50

Potter, Palmer, 28
Poussaint, Alvin, 196
primary care physicians, shortage of, 206
Pritchett, Henry, 43, 45
Provident Hospital (Baltimore), 28
Provident Hospital (Chicago), 28
Pullman, George, 28
Purvis, Charles, 14

Quillen, Jimmy, 96–97

"Race, Ethnicity, and NIH Research Awards" (Ginther), 191; *Race Traits and Tendencies of the American Negro* (Hoffman), xv–xvi
racial equality, as American principle, 198
racism: effects on NIH grant proposals, 140; heightened attention to, in 2020s, 199; in medicine, 178
Raub, William, 99
Reagan, Ronald: congresses as political backgrounds, 105–6; declining to speak at Morehouse building dedication, 114; federal budget tightening under, 75; funding cuts for disadvantaged students, 70, 114; neglect of HHS priorities, 86; support of Bob Jones University ban on interracial dating, 114
Reconstruction, post–Civil War: health disparities as legacy of, 57; refugees, post–Civil War, health crisis of, 9–10; schools established by Freedmen's Bureau, 21–22
Regan, Don, 86
Regents of the University of California v. Bakke (1978), 123
Reid, Clarice, 77
Report of the Secretary's Task Force on Black and Minority Health (Heckler Report, 1985). *See* Heckler Report
Research Centers in Minority Institutions (RCMI) program, 100–101, 136, 192, 208, 214
Research Mentoring program, NIH, 214
Reyburn, Robert, 14
Richardson, Arthur, 48, 58–59
Rock, John Swett, 24
Roentgen, Wilhelm, 40

Rogers, Paul, 65, 180
Roman, Charles, 34
root doctors, 53
Ruffin, John: building support for health disparities initiatives and research, 134–35; center of excellence designations, 169–70; conducting health disparities research across all NIH agencies, difficulties of, 173–75; constituency of, 139–40; convincing people that health disparities are real, 190; on COVID pandemic and health inequities, 200–201; as director of Office of Minority Health, 131–32; effectiveness in working with NIH institutes, 140–41; fact-finding committee on health disparities, 133–34; relationship with AMHPS, 136; Specter's support for work of, 151
Rush, Benjamin, 1–2, 39

Satcher, David: AMHPS presentation to Heckler, xix, 73–74; background and family of, 92–93; declaring smoke-free meetings for AMHPS, 68; Excellence in Minority Health Education and Care Act and, 91, 94; health disparities fact-finding committee, cochair, 134; *Journal of Health Care for the Poor and Underserved* and, 202–3; as Meharry Medical College president, 75–76, 91–92; Morehouse Medical School advisory committee and, 50; post-academic career, 184
schools, medical: AMA and professional standards for, 43; Black enrollment, male vs. female (2020), 204; costs associated with, 48–49; deficiencies, early 20th century, 42; endowments, funding for, 154–55; expansion of, 1950s–1981, 213; lack of scientific basis for US education in late 19th century, 38; NIH funding inversely associated with social mission scores, 206; Porter as advocate for Black schools, 149–50; token Black admissions in Boston schools before King's death, 72–73; white schools refusing admission

to Black students, 26; women's
medical colleges, Flexner Report
and closure of, 47. *See also names of
specific schools.*
Scott, Tim, xxi–xxii
Seven Pines, Battle of, 10
Shalala, Donna, 136, 161
Shaw University, Leonard Medical
School, 26
Shine, Kenneth, 178
Simpson, Clay, 77
Smith, James McCune: appointment to
Wilberforce University, 13;
disenrollment from Harvard
Medical School, 2; medical degree
from Glasgow University, 2;
pharmacy of, 25; rejection of Black
emigration movement, 6–7, 34–35;
relationship with Douglass, 6
Sneed, William, 23
social justice, 198, 205–6, 207, 211
social mission, of Black medical
schools, 205–6, 207
Society of Colored Physicians and
Surgeons, 34
Specter, Arlen: advocacy for medical
research, 150; as AMHPS ally, 65,
88, 104; as supporter of NIH and
medical legislation, xxi, 151
Spelman College, 55
Stanton, Edwin, 5
Starr, Paul, 45
Stevens, Rosemary, 47
Stokes, Carl, 99–100
Stokes, Louis: advocacy for health
disparities funding, xxi, 82–83, 88,
104, 127; Brain Trusts, 64–65, 90;
Disadvantaged Minority Health
Improvement Act (1990), 128–30;
on Gingrich's ferocious partisanship, 145–46; legislative achievements, 100–101, 127; productivity
of, 103–5; supporting increased
research capabilities at Black
institutions, 99–100
Straight University Medical Department, 26
Sullivan, Louis W.: afterword, 212–18;
agreement with AMHPS expansion
to non-African American communities, 208–9; AMHPS presentation

to Heckler, 73–74; avoiding conflicts of interest with AMHPS objectives, 119; chair, commission on
lack of increase in minority health
professionals, 179–80; childhood
in Blakely, Georgia, 53; desire to
return to Georgia, 59; diversity in
HHS appointments, 122–23; ethi-
cally facilitating AMHPS access to
government while HHS secretary,
125–26; as faculty member at Boston University, 48; as founding
dean, Morehouse School of Medicine, xix, 50–52; health disparities
task force membership, positive reaction to, 76–77; as HHS secretary
under George H. W. Bush, 117–19,
120–21, 122; on inadequate research capabilities at Black institutions, 99; keynote speaker at first
AMHPS biomedical symposium,
194; on lack of health care for
Blacks in 1930s, 19; Morehouse
start-up activities, 75; relationship
with George H. W. and Barbara
Bush, 116–17; retirement of, 184;
seeking public funding for Morehouse, 62–63; on shortage of minority physicians, 181, 198; social/
political change affecting AMHPS
organization, 212–13; study sections
appointments of, 125–26; testimony
on insufficient NCI spending on
minority-related research, 152
Sullivan, Walter, AMHPS biomedical
symposia and, 193–96
Sumner, Charles, 14
surgeon general, Novello replacing
Koop as, 122
Symposium on Career Opportunities
in Biomedical and Public Health
Sciences (AMHPS), 193–96

Talmadge, Herman, 65
Texas Southern University: College
of Pharmacy, xviii, 25, 64; dental
school, 25
Thompson, Tommy, 174
Thurmond, Strom, 65
Toby, Bill, 122
Tougaloo College, 13

Townsel, James, 112

Trent, William, 116

Truman, Harry, 56

Trump administration, politicized climate of, 199

Tucker, Alpheus, 14

Turner, Debbye, 195

Tuskegee College of Veterinary Medicine: AMHPS formation and, xviii, 63; center of excellence designation, 169; grants from Advanced Financial Distress Program, 92; as only predominantly Black veterinary school in US, 94

Tuskegee Institute Hospital and Nurse Training School, 28

Tyson, James, 28, 31

Unequal Treatment: Confronting Racial and Ethnic Disparities in Healthcare (Institute of Medicine), 176–79

United Negro College Fund (UNCF), 116

University of Pennsylvania Medical School, 28, 30

University of West Virginia Health System, 172

University of Würzburg, 39

US Congress: Black representatives (1968), 106; "Labor H" subcommittee and health-related funding, 145; toxic atmosphere under Gingrich, 145

US Constitution, Fourteenth Amendment, 7

US Health and Human Services Department (HHS): affiliated agencies under, 70; African American appointees to senior positions, 123–24; health of minorities neglected prior to Heckler Report, 85; Heckler as its secretary under Reagan, 70–71; reorientation on minority issues, 135; scope of, 120; Sullivan as its secretary under George H. W. Bush, 117–19

vaccines and vaccination, Black distrust of, 215–16

Varmus, Harold: director, Genome Research Institute, 187; disapproval of Research Centers in Minority Institutions program, 136; Minority Health and Health Disparities Research and Education Act opposed by, 159–62; as NIH director, 159–60, 201

Virchow, Rudolf, 39, 43

Voting Rights Act (1965), 57, 61

Warren, Rueben, 197, 202, 205–6, 207

Washington, Booker T., 94

Watts, J. C., 158

Waxman, Henry, 95–97

Welch, William Henry: family and educational background of, 38; at Johns Hopkins School of Medicine, 40–41; on lack of medical science research in US, 40; medical science studies in Germany, 39

"What If We Were Equal? A Comparison of the Black-White Mortality Gap in 1960 and 2000" (Satcher et al.), 200

White, Augustus, 177

Whitlock, Rodney, 158

Wilberforce University (Ohio), 13

Williams, Daniel Hale, 27–28, 29, 30, 33, 34

Wilson, Donald, 191

women's health, 123

Wyngaarden, James, 77, 101

Xavier University (New Orleans): College of Pharmacy, xviii, 25, 63, 64, 92; dental school, 25; history of, 95

Young, Andy, 115

Zerhouni, Elias, 174

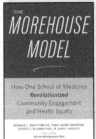
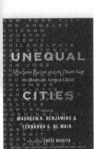
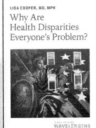
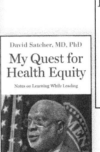
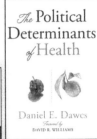
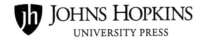

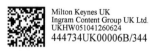